HEALTH CARE IN TRANSITION

MEDICAID AND LONG-TERM CARE ASSISTANCE

FINANCIAL ELIGIBILITY ISSUES

Health Care in Transition

Additional books in this series can be found on Nova's website under the Series tab.

Additional e-books in this series can be found on Nova's website under the e-book tab.

HEALTH CARE IN TRANSITION

MEDICAID AND LONG-TERM CARE ASSISTANCE

FINANCIAL ELIGIBILITY ISSUES

CORYNN D. FORD
EDITOR

nova publishers
New York

Library of Congress Cataloging-in-Publication Data

ISBN: 978-1-63463-328-4

Published by Nova Science Publishers, Inc. † New York

CONTENTS

PREFACE

Medicaid is a joint federal-state program that finances the delivery of primary and acute medical services, as well as LTSS, for a diverse low-income population, including children, pregnant women, adults, individuals with chronic disabling conditions, and people age 65 and older. This book describes the basic elements of Medicaid, focusing on who is eligible, what services are covered, how enrollees share in the cost of care, how the program is financed, and how providers are paid. The book also explains waivers, program integrity activities, and the dual eligible population. In addition, the book describes the following selected issues: the ACA Medicaid expansion, the impact of the ACA health insurance annual fee on Medicaid, and the ACA maintenance of effort (MOE) with respect to Medicaid eligibility.

Chapter 1 – Medicaid is a means-tested entitlement program that finances the delivery of health care and long-term services and supports (LTSS) to certain eligible low-income individuals. Established under Title XIX of the Social Security Act (SSA), the Medicaid program is state-operated within broad federal guidelines, and is jointly funded by the federal government and states. To qualify for Medicaid, individuals must meet certain *categorical* and *financial* requirements. To qualify for Medicaid LTSS, individuals must also meet state-based functional eligibility criteria. The rules for determining financial eligibility for persons who need LTSS under the Medicaid program are complex. Generally, individuals must have assets that are equal to or below established thresholds to be considered eligible for Medicaid. While these financial eligibility rules also vary by state, states must set these limits in accordance with certain federal requirements.

Under federal Medicaid law, states are required to provide coverage to aged, blind, and disabled (ABD) persons receiving cash-assistance through the

Supplemental Security Income (SSI) program. In doing so, the Medicaid program uses SSI program rules as the basis for determining financial eligibility. However, federal law gives states the option to use financial eligibility criteria that are more restrictive than SSI. States that use this alternative to SSI program rules are typically referred to as “209(b) states.” States may also extend Medicaid coverage to other population groups, referred to as optional eligibility groups. For elderly and disabled individuals potentially eligible for Medicaid LTSS coverage through these optional eligibility groups, states may use more liberal standards for determining financial eligibility than those specified under SSI program rules. Section 1902(r)(2) of the SSA gives states flexibility to modify SSI program rules with respect to counting assets (both income and resources) for the purposes of determining Medicaid eligibility. Most states use these Medicaid statutory provisions to ignore or disregard certain types of income and/or resources, thereby extending Medicaid coverage to ABD individuals with higher asset levels.

In addition, the Patient Protection and Affordable Care Act (ACA; P.L. 111-148, as amended) included the ACA Medicaid expansion, which allows states to expand Medicaid eligibility beyond the historical categorical eligibility groups to individuals under age 65 with income up to 133% of the federal poverty level (FPL) (effectively 138% FPL). In general, states are not required to offer LTSS under the ACA Medicaid expansion. However, the ACA Medicaid expansion affords states options to include LTSS or otherwise make available state plan Medicaid-covered LTSS to certain beneficiaries. As of January 1, 2014, most of Medicaid’s non-elderly populations (i.e., parents, children, pregnant women) now use modified adjusted gross income (MAGI) financial eligibility rules to determine financial eligibility for Medicaid, including those individuals eligible under the ACA Medicaid expansion.

Congress has enacted several laws over the years aimed at limiting the ability of individuals to divest financial resources in order to become eligible for Medicaid LTSS. The Tax Equity and Fiscal Responsibility Act of 1982 (TEFRA, P.L. 97-248) was the first such legislation enacted to limit the actions of individuals who divest resources for this purpose. The Omnibus Budget and Reconciliation Act of 1993 (OBRA 93, P.L. 103-66) included several provisions to restrict access to Medicaid LTSS to only those individuals who were low-income or to those who applied their assets toward the cost of their care. The Deficit Reduction Act of 2005 (DRA, P.L. 109-171) was the most recent action taken by Congress to amend the SSA by further limiting the ability of individuals to divest their assets for the purpose of qualifying for Medicaid LTSS.

This report provides an overview of the financial requirements used for determining eligibility for Medicaid LTSS. It first provides background information on the Medicaid program, including general eligibility requirements. Then it describes federal statute as well as selected regulations and guidance regarding these financial eligibility requirements, including rules related to spousal impoverishment, asset transfers, treatment of certain assets, post-eligibility treatment of income, and estate recovery.

Chapter 2 – Medicaid paid for nearly one-third of the nation's $158 billion in nursing home expenditures in 2012. To be financially eligible for Medicaid, individuals cannot have assets above certain limits. Not all assets are countable in determining Medicaid eligibility; federal law discourages individuals from reducing their countable assets, for example by transferring them to family members, to qualify for Medicaid. Although Congress has acted multiple times to address financial eligibility requirements for Medicaid coverage of nursing home care, methods exist through which individuals, sometimes with the help of attorneys, can reduce their assets and qualify for Medicaid.

GAO was asked for information on the extent to which individuals may be using available methods to qualify for Medicaid coverage. GAO (1) examined financial characteristics of applicants approved for Medicaid nursing home coverage in selected states; (2) identified methods used to reduce countable assets to qualify for Medicaid; and (3) identified information eligibility workers consider the most useful in assessing applicants' financial eligibility. GAO analyzed a random, but nongeneralizeable, sample of Medicaid nursing home applications in two counties in each of three states (Florida, New York, and South Carolina), selected based on several factors including states' asset verification efforts and demographics. GAO also interviewed officials from the Centers for Medicare & Medicaid Services, state Medicaid officials, county-based Medicaid eligibility workers, and attorneys.

Chapter 3 – Medicaid is a means-tested entitlement program that in FY2012 financed the delivery of primary and acute medical services as well as long-term services and supports to an estimated 57 million people, and cost states and the federal government $431 billion. In comparison, the Medicare program provided health care benefits to nearly 50 million seniors and certain individuals with disabilities in FY2012 at a cost of roughly $557 billion. Because Medicaid represents a large component of federal mandatory spending, Congress is likely to continue its oversight of Medicaid's eligibility, benefits, and costs.

Participation in Medicaid is voluntary for states, though all states, the District of Columbia, and U.S. territories choose to participate. In order to participate in Medicaid, the federal government requires states to cover certain mandatory populations and benefits, but the federal government also allows states to cover other optional populations and services. Due to this flexibility, there is substantial variation among the states in terms of factors such as Medicaid eligibility, covered benefits, and provider payment rates. In addition, there are several waiver and demonstration authorities that allow states to operate their Medicaid program outside of federal rules.

Historically, Medicaid eligibility has generally been limited to low-income children, pregnant women, parents of dependent children, the elderly, and individuals with disabilities; however, the Patient Protection and Affordable Care Act (ACA; P.L. 111-148, as amended) included the ACA Medicaid expansion, which expands Medicaid eligibility to individuals under the age of 65 with income up to 133% of the federal poverty level (FPL) (effectively 138% FPL) at state option.

The ACA makes a number of other changes, which together represent the most significant reform to the Medicaid program since its establishment in 1965. In addition to the ACA Medicaid expansion, the ACA also expands Medicaid eligibility for children ages 6 to 18 and former foster care children; transitions to the modified adjusted gross income (MAGI) counting methodology for most nonelderly Medicaid enrollees; requires alternative benefit plan (ABP) coverage for certain Medicaid enrollees; provides enhanced federal matching funds for the ACA Medicaid expansion; increases uniformity among Medicare, Medicaid, and the State Children's Health Insurance Program (CHIP) program integrity activities; and provides the Centers for Medicare & Medicaid Services (CMS) with the ability to test methods to improve coordination of care for dual-eligible beneficiaries, among a number of other changes.

This report describes the basic elements of Medicaid, focusing on who is eligible, what services are covered, how enrollees share in the cost of care, how the program is financed, and how providers are paid. The report also explains waivers, program integrity activities, and the dual-eligible population. In addition, the report describes the following selected issues: the ACA Medicaid expansion, the impact of the ACA health insurance annual fee on Medicaid, and the ACA maintenance of effort (MOE) with respect to Medicaid eligibility.

In: Medicaid and Long-Term Care Assistance ISBN: 978-1-63463-328-4
Editor: Corynn D. Ford

Chapter 1

MEDICAID FINANCIAL ELIGIBILITY FOR LONG-TERM SERVICES AND SUPPORTS*

Kirsten J. Colello

SUMMARY

Medicaid is a means-tested entitlement program that finances the delivery of health care and long-term services and supports (LTSS) to certain eligible low-income individuals. Established under Title XIX of the Social Security Act (SSA), the Medicaid program is state-operated within broad federal guidelines, and is jointly funded by the federal government and states. To qualify for Medicaid, individuals must meet certain *categorical* and *financial* requirements. To qualify for Medicaid LTSS, individuals must also meet state-based functional eligibility criteria. The rules for determining financial eligibility for persons who need LTSS under the Medicaid program are complex. Generally, individuals must have assets that are equal to or below established thresholds to be considered eligible for Medicaid. While these financial eligibility rules also vary by state, states must set these limits in accordance with certain federal requirements.

Under federal Medicaid law, states are required to provide coverage to aged, blind, and disabled (ABD) persons receiving cash-assistance through the Supplemental Security Income (SSI) program. In doing so,

* This is an edited, reformatted and augmented version of a Congressional Research Service publication R43506, prepared for Members and Committees of Congress, dated April 24, 2014.

the Medicaid program uses SSI program rules as the basis for determining financial eligibility. However, federal law gives states the option to use financial eligibility criteria that are more restrictive than SSI. States that use this alternative to SSI program rules are typically referred to as "209(b) states." States may also extend Medicaid coverage to other population groups, referred to as optional eligibility groups. For elderly and disabled individuals potentially eligible for Medicaid LTSS coverage through these optional eligibility groups, states may use more liberal standards for determining financial eligibility than those specified under SSI program rules. Section 1902(r)(2) of the SSA gives states flexibility to modify SSI program rules with respect to counting assets (both income and resources) for the purposes of determining Medicaid eligibility. Most states use these Medicaid statutory provisions to ignore or disregard certain types of income and/or resources, thereby extending Medicaid coverage to ABD individuals with higher asset levels.

In addition, the Patient Protection and Affordable Care Act (ACA; P.L. 111-148, as amended) included the ACA Medicaid expansion, which allows states to expand Medicaid eligibility beyond the historical categorical eligibility groups to individuals under age 65 with income up to 133% of the federal poverty level (FPL) (effectively 138% FPL). In general, states are not required to offer LTSS under the ACA Medicaid expansion. However, the ACA Medicaid expansion affords states options to include LTSS or otherwise make available state plan Medicaid-covered LTSS to certain beneficiaries. As of January 1, 2014, most of Medicaid's non-elderly populations (i.e., parents, children, pregnant women) now use modified adjusted gross income (MAGI) financial eligibility rules to determine financial eligibility for Medicaid, including those individuals eligible under the ACA Medicaid expansion.

Congress has enacted several laws over the years aimed at limiting the ability of individuals to divest financial resources in order to become eligible for Medicaid LTSS. The Tax Equity and Fiscal Responsibility Act of 1982 (TEFRA, P.L. 97-248) was the first such legislation enacted to limit the actions of individuals who divest resources for this purpose. The Omnibus Budget and Reconciliation Act of 1993 (OBRA 93, P.L. 103-66) included several provisions to restrict access to Medicaid LTSS to only those individuals who were low-income or to those who applied their assets toward the cost of their care. The Deficit Reduction Act of 2005 (DRA, P.L. 109-171) was the most recent action taken by Congress to amend the SSA by further limiting the ability of individuals to divest their assets for the purpose of qualifying for Medicaid LTSS.

This report provides an overview of the financial requirements used for determining eligibility for Medicaid LTSS. It first provides background information on the Medicaid program, including general eligibility requirements. Then it describes federal statute as well as selected regulations and guidance regarding these financial eligibility requirements, including rules related to spousal impoverishment, asset transfers, treatment of certain assets, post-eligibility treatment of income, and estate recovery.

INTRODUCTION

Long-term services and supports (LTSS) refer to a broad range of health and health-related services and supports needed by individuals who lack the capacity for self-care due to a physical, cognitive, or mental disability or condition. Often the individual's disability or condition results in the need for hands-on assistance or supervision over an extended period of time. LTSS includes services provided in institutional settings such as nursing homes as well as services provided in home and community-based residential settings such as private homes or assisted living facilities.

The cost of obtaining paid LTSS may far exceed many individuals' financial resources. In 2014, the median annual cost of nursing home care was just over $77,000 for a semi-private room and almost $88,000 for a private room.[1] For those receiving paid LTSS at home, the cost for these services can vary depending on the amount and duration of care provided. Assuming 18 hours of care per week, the median annual cost of home health aide services would have been over $19,000 in 2014.[2] Large personal financial liabilities associated with paying for LTSS may leave some individuals and their families at financial risk. As a result, some individuals may turn to public programs for assistance with the high costs of needed LTSS.

Medicaid is a means-tested entitlement program that finances the delivery of health care and LTSS to certain eligible low-income individuals. Established under Title XIX of the Social Security Act (SSA), the Medicaid program is state-operated within broad federal guidelines, and is jointly funded by the federal government and states. Medicaid is also the largest payer of LTSS in the United States. In 2012, the program paid 42.0% of all LTSS expenditures at $136.3 billion, out of a total of $324.2 billion.[3] LTSS expenditures also represent a significant portion of total Medicaid expenditures, comprising more than one-third (35.3%) of the total spent on Medicaid in that year. The most recent data available estimated that 4.2 million Medicaid beneficiaries (or 6.4%) of the 60 million total enrolled Medicaid population received LTSS in 2010, accounting for over one-third of the costs.[4] Some states are reexamining their Medicaid programs in an effort to control state LTSS spending.

Historically, Medicaid has covered LTSS for individuals who are unable to afford the cost of their care. Moreover, federal and state governments have a financial interest in ensuring that only eligible individuals receive Medicaid coverage for LTSS. In response, Congress has enacted several laws over the years aimed at limiting the ability of individuals to divest financial resources in an effort to protect them (e.g., preserve them for a family member), thereby meeting financial requirements for Medicaid and any applicable LTSS. The Tax Equity and Fiscal Responsibility Act of 1982 (TEFRA, P.L. 97-248) was the first such legislation enacted to limit the actions of individuals who divest resources for this purpose. The Omnibus Budget and Reconciliation Act of 1993 (OBRA 93, P.L. 103-66) included several provisions to restrict access to Medicaid LTSS to only those individuals who were low-income or to those who applied their financial resources toward the cost of their care. The Deficit Reduction Act of 2005 (DRA, P.L. 109-171) was the most recent action taken by Congress to amend the SSA by further limiting the ability of individuals to divest their resources for the purpose of qualifying for Medicaid LTSS.

This report provides an overview of the financial requirements used for determining eligibility for Medicaid LTSS. It first provides background information on the Medicaid program, including general eligibility requirements. Next, it describes federal statute as well as selected regulations and guidance regarding these financial eligibility requirements, including rules related to spousal impoverishment, asset transfers, treatment of certain assets, post-eligibility treatment of income, and estate recovery.

MEDICAID FINANCIAL ELIGIBILITY FOR LONG-TERM SERVICES AND SUPPORTS

Eligibility for Medicaid is determined by both federal and state law, whereby states set individual eligibility criteria within federal minimum standards. Individuals must meet *categorical* (e.g., individuals aged 65 and over, individuals with disabilities, children, pregnant women, parents, certain nonelderly childless adults) and *financial* (i.e., income and sometimes resource limits) criteria. The categorical groups most often associated with the need for Medicaid-covered LTSS are the aged, blind, and disabled (ABD). Individuals must also meet other non-financial eligibility criteria, including federal and state residency requirements, immigration status, and documentation of U.S. citizenship. In addition to categorical and financial eligibility criteria, individuals in need of Medicaid-covered LTSS must also meet state-based functional eligibility criteria.[5]

Federal Medicaid law requires states to cover certain population groups (mandatory eligibility groups) and gives states the flexibility to cover other population groups (optional eligibility groups).[6] The Patient Protection and Affordable Care Act (ACA; P.L. 111-148, as amended) included the ACA Medicaid expansion, which, at state option, extends Medicaid eligibility beyond the historical categorical eligibility groups to individuals under age 65 with income up to 133% of the federal poverty level (FPL), effectively 138% FPL (after adjusting for a 5% income disregard for individuals at the highest income limits for coverage).[7]

The rules for determining financial eligibility for individuals who need Medicaid-covered LTSS are complex. Eligibility for the program's benefits has traditionally been linked to eligibility for cash assistance programs. For example, under federal Medicaid law, states are required to provide coverage to ABD individuals receiving cash-assistance through the Supplemental Security Income (SSI) program. In doing so, the Medicaid program uses SSI program rules as the basis for determining financial eligibility. However, federal law gives states the option to use financial eligibility criteria that are more restrictive than SSI.[8] These SSI coverage requirements are referred to as the SSI-related mandatory eligibility groups. For 2014, the SSI rules specify that recipients must have monthly income at or below $721 for an individual (or $1,082 for a couple), about 75% of the federal poverty level (FPL).[9] SSI rules also limit the countable resources individuals may have to $2,000 for an individual (or $3,000 for a couple).[10]

States may also extend Medicaid coverage to other ABD individuals, referred to as optional eligibility groups. For ABD individuals potentially eligible for Medicaid through these optional eligibility groups, states may use SSI program rules or they may use more liberal standards for determining financial eligibility than those specified under SSI.[11] Most states use these Medicaid statutory provisions to ignore or disregard certain types of income and/or resources, thereby extending Medicaid eligibility to ABD individuals with higher asset levels. For example, states may extend Medicaid coverage to individuals who have income up to three times the basic SSI payment level (referred to as the 300% rule) and reside in a nursing facility or other institution. Medicaid also provides states the option of covering elderly and disabled persons who are not poor by SSI standards but who need assistance with medical expenses. Under the medically needy pathway, individuals can qualify for Medicaid if they have income and resources that exceed the standards established by the states for the medically needy programs, but only if they incur medical expenses that "spend-down" or deplete their income and resources to specified levels.

In contrast, the rules for determining financial eligibility for most of Medicaid's non-elderly population (i.e., parents, children, pregnant women) use modified adjusted gross income (MAGI). These MAGI rules also apply to those individuals eligible under the ACA Medicaid expansion.[12] In this report, individuals who are determined eligible for Medicaid using MAGI rules are collectively referred to as "MAGI individuals." There are no additional resource requirements used to determine Medicaid financial eligibility for MAGI individuals (i.e., no resource limit). According to CMS, in ACA Medicaid expansion states individuals under age 65 with disabilities who have LTSS needs are likely to continue to qualify for Medicaid under optional eligibility groups related to disability.[13,14] These "non-MAGI individuals" are still subject to the financial eligibility rules associated with those eligibility groups (i.e., both income and resource limits). Nevertheless, some adults with disabilities who need LTSS may still qualify and receive Medicaid-covered LTSS under the ACA Medicaid expansion. These individuals would be subject to MAGI financial eligibility rules (i.e., income limit, but no resource limit). For example, individuals who meet the categorical requirements for disabled and have income under 138% FPL but resources above the level required to otherwise qualify through other optional groups may be eligible under the Medicaid ACA expansion.

In general, states are not required to offer LTSS for individuals in the ACA Medicaid expansion group. However, the ACA Medicaid expansion affords states options to include LTSS or otherwise make available state plan Medicaid-covered LTSS to certain newly eligible enrollees. States that chose to implement the ACA Medicaid expansion are required to provide coverage through Alternative Benefit Plans (ABPs), which must include the 10 essential health benefits (EHBs). However, specific groups are exempt from mandatory enrollment in ABPs (e.g., those with special health care needs such as disabling mental disorders or serious and complex medical conditions). These individuals must be offered the option of a benefit plan that includes Medicaid state plan services.[15] For most adult beneficiaries receiving state plan services, they may be eligible for certain mandatory LTSS (e.g., nursing facility services, home health services) and optional state plan LTSS (e.g., personal care services). In addition, some states may choose to include LTSS in their ABPs.

Prior to the ACA Medicaid expansion, eligibility pathways available to adults with disabilities in need of LTSS required both income and resource limits. Under the ACA Medicaid expansion, adults with disabilities may be able to receive LTSS without specified resource limits. For these MAGI Individuals to potentially retain financial resources that could be applied toward the cost of their care raises beneficiary equity issues within the Medicaid program. On February 19, 2014, CMS released guidance to states on how the LTSS-related resource rules apply to MAGI individuals.[16] This information is included in the report, where applicable.

General Asset Rules

Assessment of an applicant's assets for the purposes of determining Medicaid eligibility can be complicated, depending on how much and what type of assets an individual possesses. Under the Medicaid program, assets fall into one of two categories: (1) income or (2) resources. In general, income includes *earned* income such as wages, self-employment earnings, and royalties, as well as *unearned* income, which includes payments from annuities, pensions, and trusts. Resources are generally defined as cash and other liquid assets or personal property that an individual (or a spouse) owns and could convert to cash.[17] States have the flexibility to determine income and resource requirements for different Medicaid eligibility groups within broad federal guidelines. For the SSI-related mandatory eligibility groups, states rely on SSI program rules for determining financial eligibility, with options to use more restrictive requirements in 209(b) states. States have further flexibility to modify SSI program rules in determining income and resource requirements for other optional eligibility groups.

Under SSI program rules, resources may be (1) counted based on their entire value, (2) excluded for their entire value, or (3) excluded for part of their value.[18] Resources that are counted for their entire value generally include liquid assets that the applicant owns and could convert to cash (e.g., money in bank accounts, stocks and bonds, mutual fund investments, and certificates of deposit). Resources excluded for their entire value include a primary residence, personal and household items (e.g., furniture, appliances, personal computers, personal jewelry, personal care items, or items of cultural or religious significance), certain property essential to income-producing activity, and the value of a burial space. Further, one automobile, regardless of value, is excluded so long as it is used for transportation of the applicant or a member of the applicant's household. Resources that are excluded for part of their value include burial funds and the "face value" of certain life insurance policies (up to $1,500).[19]

Home Equity Rule

While a primary residence, regardless of value, is not a countable resource for the purposes of Medicaid eligibility under SSI program rules, the equity value of a home may affect whether or not an individual receives Medicaid covered LTSS. For beneficiaries applying for Medicaid coverage for nursing facility services or home and community-based services, federal Medicaid law restricts eligibility if the applicant's equity interest in the home exceeds a statutorily determined amount ($543,000 in 2014).[20] At state option, this threshold could be higher (up to $814,000 in 2013).[21] Such thresholds do not apply to individuals who have a spouse, child under the age of 21, or a child with a disability of any age residing in the home. Also, states can choose not to apply this rule if it is determined that doing so would cause an undue hardship in a given case. Similarly, MAGI individuals whose home equity exceeds the state threshold are not eligible for LTSS coverage.[22]

For purposes of qualifying for Medicaid LTSS, individuals who have home equity above the state-specified threshold could use a reverse mortgage or home equity loan to reduce their total equity interest in the home. In order for the proceeds of a reverse mortgage or home equity loan to be excluded from countable resources for the purposes of obtaining Medicaid coverage, federal guidance specifies that the Medicaid applicant must either spend the transaction amount or repay it to the lender in the month received.[23] Any amounts not spent or repaid in the following month are counted as resources against the state's threshold; therefore, the amount would have to be depleted before qualifying for Medicaid LTSS.

Spousal Impoverishment Protections

Adding to the complexity of determining financial eligibility for Medicaid LTSS is the treatment of the assets of a couple, when one spouse needs institutional care (the institutional spouse) and the other is able to remain in the community (the community spouse). Medicaid specifies rules for equitably allocating how much income and resources, as well as which resources, are to be credited to each spouse for the purposes of determining Medicaid LTSS eligibility. Commonly referred to as *spousal impoverishment* rules, they are intended to prevent the impoverishment of the spouse remaining in the community.[24] In general, states must establish minimum income and resource allowances within federal limits that a community spouse may hold that may not be applied toward the institutional spouse's Medicaid eligibility determination or LTSS costs.

Regarding income, federal Medicaid law exempts all of a community spouse's income in his or her name from being considered available to the other spouse. That is, for any month the institutionalized spouse is residing in an institution, income solely attributable to the community spouse is not considered available to the institutionalized spouse.[25] For community spouses with limited income, federal law allows institutionalized spouses to transfer income to the community spouse up to a state-determined minimum monthly income threshold, referred to as the minimum monthly maintenance needs allowance, that is set within federal limits. In 2014, the community spouse's minimum monthly maintenance needs allowance must be at least $1,939, but no more than $2,931, as determined by the state.[26] Following a hearing requested by either the institutionalized or community spouse, states may raise the minimum amount on income that a community spouse may retain in cases of severe hardship. Finally, Medicaid provides for additional income allowances for excess housing costs and when dependents live with the community spouse.[27]

In terms of resources, federal Medicaid law allows states to select the amount of resources a community spouse may be allowed to retain within federal limits. For 2014, this threshold must be at least $23,448 but no more than $117,240.[28] For purposes of determining the amount of resources the community spouse can retain, all resources of the couple are combined, counted, and split in half, regardless of which of the two spouses has ownership of the individual resources. If the community spouse's resources are less than the state threshold, then the Medicaid applicant must transfer his or her share of the resources to the community spouse until the community spouse's share reaches the threshold. All other non-exempt resources tied to the applicant must be depleted before the applicant can qualify for Medicaid. Similar to the treatment of income, no resources of the community spouse are considered available to the institutionalized spouse once the institutionalized spouse is determined to be eligible for Medicaid.

Prior to enactment of the ACA, spousal impoverishment rules applied only in situations where the Medicaid recipient was receiving LTSS in an institutional setting, such as a nursing facility. Section 2404 of the ACA requires states to extend spousal impoverishment rules to beneficiaries receiving certain home and community-based services (HCBS).[29] Beginning in 2014, the expansion of spousal impoverishment rules apply to individuals who (1) receive HCBS through SSA waiver authorities such as Section 1115 Research and Demonstration waivers, Section 1915(c) HCBS waivers, and the Section 1915(d) HCBS waivers for the elderly; (2) receive services through the Section 1915(i) state plan amendment option to provide HCBS; (3) are determined "medically needy";[30] or (4) receive personal attendant services under the Community First Choice Option under Section 1915(k).[31] This provision remains in effect for the five-year period beginning on January 1, 2014.

Asset Transfers

For persons seeking Medicaid LTSS eligibility, federal Medicaid law requires states to apply rules regarding the transfer of assets prior to qualifying for Medicaid.[32] These rules attempt to ensure that Medicaid applicants apply their assets toward the cost of their care and do not divest them to gain Medicaid eligibility sooner than would occur otherwise. Specifically, Medicaid may require states to delay Medicaid eligibility for applicants seeking institutional and certain home and community-based LTSS who have disposed of certain assets for less than fair market value (FMV) on or after a "look-back" period, or period of time prior to application for services. This look-back period is five years prior to application for Medicaid. [33] In other words, transfers for less than FMV may be, but are not always, prohibited during the five-year period prior to application for Medicaid. Federal Medicaid law also prohibits spouses of applicants from transferring assets for less than FMV during this same period. These asset transfer rules apply to MAGI individuals who seek coverage for Medicaid LTSS.[34]

In order to determine whether a transfer for less than FMV occurred, applicants are first asked whether they made any transfers of monetary value during the five-year "look-back" period. If at least one transfer has occurred during this period, the state must determine whether the transfer was made for FMV. If the transfer was made for less than FMV (often referred to as an improper transfer), a penalty is imposed on the applicant in the form of months of ineligibility. To calculate the penalty period, the monetary value of the transfer, or portion of the transfer, that was made for less than FMV is divided by the average monthly private pay rate for nursing facility services in the state (or at state option, the rate in the community in which the individual resides). For example, an improper transfer of $20,000 divided by an average monthly private pay rate in a nursing facility of $5,000 results in a four-month period of ineligibility for Medicaid LTSS.

The penalty period begins either on the first day of the month in which assets have been transferred for less than FMV, or the date on which the individual is eligible for Medicaid and would otherwise be receiving an institutional level of care, whichever is later. In addition, states may waive penalties for asset transfers if the applicant can demonstrate to the state that he or she either (1) intended to transfer assets for FMV; (2) transferred assets for a purpose other than to qualify for medical assistance; or (3) recovered the assets that had been previously transferred. Also, ineligibility for Medicaid coverage is limited to certain LTSS, and individuals may still be eligible for other Medicaid services.[35]

Not all asset transfers during the five-year look back period are subject to penalties.[36] For example, asset transfers for FMV, transfers to spouses of any value, and certain transfers to other individuals, such as children with disabilities, are not subject to penalties. Also, a home may be excluded from asset transfer penalties if it is transferred to certain individuals, including a spouse, a child under the age of 21, a child who is blind or permanently and totally disabled, or a son or daughter who has resided in the home for at least two years immediately before the date the individual enters an institutional facility and has provided care that permitted the individual to delay institutionalization. These rules are intended to ensure that certain family members would not be without housing or lose their homes in order for another family member to obtain Medicaid coverage.

Treatment of Certain Types of Assets

For the purposes of Medicaid asset transfer rules, all resources (and income) of an individual or couple are evaluated to determine whether the establishment, purchase, sale, or transfer of an asset has occurred for less than FMV. Generally, states follow SSI program rules concerning the treatment of most asset types that individuals possess at the time of application to Medicaid. Although Medicaid law does not contain provisions specifying how *all* assets should be treated, it does include special rules about how states must treat *certain* types of assets, such as annuities, fees for Continuing Care

Retirement Communities (CCRCs), life estates, promissory notes, loans, mortgages, and trusts. Also, the Secretary of the Department of Health and Human Services (HHS) has the authority to issue guidance to states on other categories of transactions that may be treated as transfers of assets for less than FMV. States must apply the rules relating to these transactions to MAGI individuals in the same way they are applied to non-MAGI individuals.[37]

Annuities

An annuity is a financial product that provides the investor with the right to receive fixed, periodic payments, either for life or for a specified term of years. For the purposes of determining Medicaid eligibility, federal Medicaid law describes when annuities should be treated as countable resources and when they should not.[38] In general, annuities are treated as transfers for less than FMV, and thus subject to penalties, except when the state is named as a beneficiary of the annuity for at least the amounts paid by Medicaid for certain LTSS (or as a secondary beneficiary after the community spouse, or minor or disabled child and such spouse or representative of the child does not dispose of the remainder of the annuity for less than FMV). Certain annuities may be excluded from penalties if they (1) are irrevocable and non-assignable, actuarially sound, and provide for payments in equal amounts during the term of the annuity (with no deferral and no balloon payments); or (2) fall into certain categories specified in Section 408 of the Internal Revenue Service Code of 1986 (IRC). Annuities that are defined as individual retirement accounts under federal tax code or purchased with the proceeds of certain retirement accounts and meet certain federal tax code requirements are not considered transfers for less than FMV if purchased by or on the behalf of an individual who applied for Medicaid coverage for LTSS.

Individuals seeking Medicaid LTSS are required to submit a financial disclosure statement of any interest the individual (or community spouse, if applicable) has in an annuity or similar financial product, regardless of whether the annuity meets the criteria for exclusion from countable resources.[39] All annuities are penalized as transfers for less than FMV if the applicant fails to file the necessary disclosure documentation from the financial institution, employer, or employer association that issued the annuity.[40]

Fees for Continuing Care Retirement Communities

Continuing Care Retirement Communities (CCRCs) or life care communities offer a range of housing and services, including LTSS, to older individuals as their care needs change over time. Generally, CCRCs provide housing with various levels of LTSS arrangements such as independent living, assisted living, and nursing facility care. CCRCs are paid primarily with private funds, but a number also accept Medicaid payments for certain services, such as nursing facility care. Residents of CCRCs or life care communities are required to spend their resources, declared when applying for admission, on their care before they apply for Medicaid. Federal Medicaid law requires states to consider certain entrance fees for CCRCs or life care communities as countable resources for the purposes of determining an individual's eligibility for Medicaid.[41]

Life Estates

Generally, a life estate entitles an individual to possess, use, and obtain profits from a property for as long as he or she lives, even though the actual ownership of the property has passed on to another. For example, an individual may transfer home ownership to a son or daughter, but retain the use of the home throughout their lifetime. Such a transaction would give the child a "remainder interest" in the home, while the older individuals retained a "life estate." Upon death, the title of the home automatically passes on to the son or daughter without the need for probate. With respect to Medicaid asset transfer rules, the purchase of a life estate is considered a transfer for less than FMV, and subject to an asset transfer penalty, when the value of the transferred property is greater that the value of the rights conferred by the life estate.[42] The purchase of a life estate is also considered a transfer of assets for less than FMV unless the purchaser resides in the home for at least one year after the date of purchase.[43]

Promissory Notes, Loans, and Mortgages

Funds used to purchase a promissory note, loan, or mortgage are considered a transfer of assets for less than FMV unless the repayment terms are (1) actuarially sound; (2) provide for payments to be made in equal amounts during the term of the loan (with no deferral or balloon payments); and (3) prohibit the cancellation of the balance upon the death of the lender.[44] Should the promissory note, loan, or mortgage not satisfy the above requirements, the penalty amount is the amount of the outstanding balance due at the time the individual applies for Medicaid.

Trusts

Most trusts are considered assets available to the individual for the cost of their care, and, if transferred, could be considered assets that have been transferred for less than FMV.[45] An individual is considered to have established a trust if the individual's assets were used to form all or part of the trust and if certain persons established the trust, including the individual, the individual's spouse, or a person with legal authority to act on behalf of the individual or spouse. Medicaid law establishes rules for the treatment of assets in two types of trusts: *revocable* and *irrevocable*.

A *revocable* trust can be altered after it is established (i.e., assets may be added or new beneficiaries may be named), whereas an *irrevocable* trust cannot be altered once it is established. In the case of a *revocable* trust, the assets used to establish the trust are deemed resources available to the individual. Payments from the trust to or for the benefit of the individual must be considered income of the individual. Any other payments from the trust are considered assets disposed of by the individual and subject to asset transfer rules. In the case of an *irrevocable* trust, if there are any circumstances under which payments can be made from the trust for the benefit of the individual, then the assets used to establish the trust and payments from the trust are considered income and resources of the individual. Any other payments from the trust are considered assets disposed of by the individual and subject to asset transfer rules. An irrevocable trust from which no portion of the trust could be considered payment to the individual shall be subject to asset transfer rules, as of the date of the trust's establishment or date on which payment occurred, whichever is later. States are required to establish procedures for waiving the application of these rules in cases of undue hardship.

Post-Eligibility Treatment of Income

Medicaid has another set of rules for the treatment of income after a person has become eligible for coverage and is either living in an institution, such as a nursing facility, or is receiving Section 1915(c) HCBS waiver services while living in the community. These rules are commonly referred to as the *post-eligibility treatment of income* (PETI) rules. In general, beneficiaries qualifying through certain eligibility groups are required to apply their income exceeding specified amounts toward the cost of their care. Within federal guidelines, a beneficiary may retain a certain amount of income for personal use based on the services one receives. The amounts a beneficiary may retain vary by care setting.

For beneficiaries receiving Medicaid LTSS in an institutional facility, a monthly personal needs allowance (PNA) is permitted.[46] The PNA is an amount that is considered reasonable to cover various personal care items not included in the institution's basic charge. Beneficiaries may retain a monthly PNA from their income for clothing and other personal expenses. The beneficiary then applies the remainder of his or her income toward the cost of care. When receiving nursing facility services, Medicaid statute requires states to allow individuals to retain a minimum PNA of at least $30 per month for an institutionalized individual, though the amount can be higher and varies by state.

For beneficiaries living in the community and enrolled in Section 1915(c) HCBS waivers, a monthly maintenance needs allowance (MMNA) is permitted.[47] The MMNA is an amount that is considered reasonable to cover various living expenses in the community. Beneficiaries may retain an MMNA from their income for housing, food, and other personal expenses. The beneficiary then applies the rest of his or her income toward the cost of care. Federal regulations require states to set a maximum amount for the MMNA based on a reasonable assessment of need.[48] In 2009, the most recent year for which data are available, this amount ranged from $600 to $2,022 per month across states.[49]

CMS guidance regarding the application of PETI rules to MAGI individuals states that such rules are limited to certain eligibility groups that rely on the financial methodologies from the SSI and former Aid to Families with Dependent Children (AFDC) cash assistance programs. Thus, these post-eligibilty rules do not apply to Medicaid beneficiaries whose eligibility is based on MAGI methodologies. CMS states that the statute provides authority to "expand the reach" of the post-eligibility regulations to include MAGI individuals who receive LTSS coverage as there are "equity reasons to consider the application of these rules to MAGI individuals." [50]Accordingly, the agency is considering rulemaking on this issue.

ESTATE RECOVERY

Other provisions in Medicaid seek to recover Medicaid costs through estate recovery programs. Federal Medicaid law requires states to recover from beneficiary estates any amounts paid for certain LTSS and other related services upon a beneficiary's death.[51] Specifically, states are required to pursue the estates of

- individuals receiving services in a nursing facility or intermediate care facility for the developmentally disabled (ICF/DD), regardless of age upon the sale of property subject to a lien, and
- individuals aged 55 and older who received Medicaid assistance in nursing facilities, HCBS, and related hospital and prescription drug services.

States also have the option to recover funds spent on other items or services covered under the Medicaid state plan for individuals aged 55 and older.

Estate recovery is limited to the amounts paid by Medicaid for services received by an individual and is limited to only those assets owned by the beneficiary at the time of recovery. As a result, estate recovery is generally applied to a beneficiary's home, if available, and certain other assets within a beneficiary's estate. For purposes of these estate recovery requirements, Medicaid statute defines an estate as all real and personal property subject to a state's probate law. Under certain circumstances, annuities are included in this definition.[52] States may expand the definition of estate to include other real or personal property and other assets to which the Medicaid beneficiary has legal title or interest at the time of death.[53] Estate recovery may be made only after the death of the individual and his or her surviving spouse, if any, and only at a time when there is neither a surviving child under age 21 nor a child, of any age, who is blind or permanently and totally disabled.

To aid in estate recovery, states are authorized to impose liens on the property of certain beneficiaries prior to or after the beneficiary's death.[54] Liens may be imposed only when the individual resides in a nursing facility, ICF/DD, or other medical institution determined by the state; after notice of and opportunity for a hearing is given; and it is determined that the individual cannot reasonably be expected to return to the home. Liens may also be placed on property when, based on a court's judgment, Medicaid payments have been improperly paid on behalf of the individual. States are prohibited from pursuing liens under certain circumstances. For example, the state cannot place a lien on an individual's home if any of the following individuals reside in the home: a surviving spouse; a child under the age of 21 or a blind or permanently disabled child of any age; or a sibling of the individual who has equity interest in the property and has resided in the home at least one year prior to the individual entering an institution. Medicaid law also requires states to dissolve any lien placed on a home if the individual is discharged from the institution and returns home. In addition, liens can apply only to beneficiaries receiving institutional care who are also subject to the post-eligibility treatment of income (PETI) rules described in the previous section. Thus, liens cannot be applied to MAGI individuals who are not subject to PETI rules. However, as previously mentioned, CMS is considering rulemaking to expand PETI rules to include MAGI individuals who receive LTSS coverage.[55]

Furthermore, federal Medicaid law provides for exemptions from estate recovery in situations when such recovery would create undue hardship. Medicaid guidance allows for state flexibility in establishing procedures for an undue hardship waiver.[56] In addition to exemptions for undue hardship, Medicaid permits states to forgo estate recovery in cases where it would not be costeffective.[57] Federal Medicaid law also prohibits estate recovery in cases when a lien has been placed on the home when certain individuals reside in the home. Such instances include (1) a sibling of an individual who has resided in the home at least one year prior to the individual entering an institution, and (2) an adult child who has resided in the home for at least two years prior to the parent's institutionalization, has resided there continuously since that time, and can establish to the state's satisfaction that the adult child provided care to the parent that delayed the need for nursing facility services. Special provisions apply to persons who become eligible for Medicaid under a more liberal asset standard used in certain states for those who purchase longterm care insurance.[58]

MAGI individuals who were 55 years of age or older when they received Medicaid benefits are not exempt from these estate recovery provisions; however, the above exemptions from estate recovery also apply. In guidance issued on February 21, 2014, CMS states that Medicaid estate recovery may create a potential barrier to enrollment for some newly eligible individuals in ACA Medicaid expansion states. The guidance further articulates the agency's intention to explore options and use existing authorities to eliminate estate recovery for MAGI individuals who receive Medicaid benefits other than LTSS. CMS also notes that states have existing authority to limit the scope of estate recovery to Medicaid beneficiaries 55 and older who receive LTSS.[59]

End Notes

[1] Genworth Financial, Genworth 2014 Cost of Care Survey: Home Care Providers, Adult Day Health Care Facilities, Assisted Living Facilities and Nursing Homes, 2014.

[2] Ibid.

[3] CRS analysis of National Health Expenditure Account (NHEA) data obtained from the Centers for Medicare & Medicaid Services (CMS), Office of the Actuary, prepared December 3, 2013.

[4] Medicaid and CHIP Payment and Access Commission (MACPAC), Report to the Congress on Medicaid and CHIP, June 14, 2013, pg. 102.

[5] To define level-of-care criteria, states may use "functional" criteria such as an individual's ability to perform certain Activities of Daily Living (ADLs, e.g., eating, bathing, dressing, and walking) or to perform certain Instrumental Activities of Daily Living (IADLs, e.g., shopping, housework, and meal preparation) that allow an individual to live independently in the community. Other states may use "clinical" level-of-care criteria that include diagnosis of an illness, injury, disability or other medical condition, treatment and medications, and cognitive status, among other information. Most states use a combination of functional and clinical criteria in defining the need for LTSS. For further information on state specific level-of-care criteria, see L. Hendrickson and G. Kyzr-Sheeley, "Determining Medicaid Nursing Home Eligibility: A Survey of State Level of Care Assessment," Rutgers Center for State Health Policy, March 2008.

[6] For more information, see CRS Report R43357, Medicaid: An Overview, coordinated by Alison Mitchell.

[7] On June 28, 2012, the U.S. Supreme Court issued a decision in National Federation of Independent Business v. Sebelius. The Court held that the federal government cannot terminate current Medicaid program federal matching funds if a state does not expand its Medicaid program, effectively making the ACA Medicaid expansion for this new "adult" group optional.

[8] States that use this alternative to SSI program rules are typically referred to as "209(b) states," which refers to the statutory authority in the Social Security Amendments of 1972 (SSA 72, P.L. 92-603) that allows states to use more restrictive eligibility criteria than the SSI program, but no more restrictive than those criteria in effect on January 1, 1972. In these states, SSI receipt does not guarantee Medicaid eligibility. There are 11 209(b) states: Connecticut, Hawaii, Illinois, Indiana, Minnesota, Missouri, New Hampshire, North Dakota, Ohio, Oklahoma, and Virginia.

[9] CMS, 2014 SSI and Spousal Impoverishment Standards, http://www.medicaid.gov/Medicaid-CHIP-ProgramInformation/By-Topics/Eligibility/Downloads/Spousal-Impoverishment-2014.pdf

[10] The SSI resource limit is not subject to annual increases and has not changed since 1989.

[11] Section 1902(r)(2) of the SSA gives states flexibility to modify SSI program rules with respect to counting assets for the purposes of determining Medicaid eligibility.

[12] MAGI is defined as the Internal Revenue Code's adjusted gross income (AGI, which reflects a number of deductions, including trade and business deductions, losses from sale of property, and alimony payments) increased (if applicable) by tax-exempt interest and income earned by U.S. citizens or residents living abroad. For more information, see CRS Report R41997, Definition of Income for Certain Medicaid Provisions and Premium Credits in ACA, coordinated by Christine Scott.

[13] State Medicaid Directors Letter SMDL#14-001, ACA #29, Centers for Medicare & Medicaid Services, Department of Health and Human Services, February 21, 2014, http://www.medicaid.gov/Federal-Policy-Guidance/Downloads/ SMD-14-001.pdf.

[14] In addition, CMS regulations enable individuals with disabilities who may need LTSS and are eligible under the ACA Medicaid expansion, as well as other optional eligibility pathways, to choose to enroll under an optional eligibility pathway which better meets their needs.

Centers for Medicare & Medicaid Services, "Medicaid Program; Eligibility Changes Under the Affordable Care Act of 2010," 77 Federal Register 17194 and 17208, March 23, 2012.

[15] For a discussion of Medicaid coverage of LTSS and alternative benefit plans (ABPs), see CRS Report R43328, Medicaid Coverage of Long Term Services and Supports, by Kirsten J. Colello, pp. 10-11.

[16] Ibid.

[17] 20 CFR 416.1201.

[18] Section 1613 of the SSA specifies items that are excluded from resource counting rules. Federal regulation 20 CFR 416.1210 further clarifies under what conditions resources may be excluded.

[19] Life insurance is counted as a resource to the extent of its cash surrender value. If the total face value of all life insurance policies does not exceed $1,500, no part of the cash surrender value is considered. In determining the face value of life insurance, term insurance and burial insurance are not considered (20 CFR 416.1230).

[20] The equity interest in a home is the fair market value of the home (i.e., what an individual could sell the home for on the open market) minus the amount of any outstanding debts, such as a mortgage or home equity loan.

[21] Section 1917(f) of the SSA. Through 2010, federal law limited eligibility for Medicaid LTSS if the applicant's equity interest in the home was greater than $500,000. At state option, this threshold could be as high as $750,000. Starting in 2011, these thresholds increase each year based on the percentage increase in the consumer price index for all urban consumers (CPI-U), rounded to the nearest $1,000.

[22] State Medicaid Directors Letter SMDL#14-001, ACA #29, Centers for Medicare & Medicaid Services, Department of Health and Human Services, February 21, 2014, http://www.medicaid.gov/Federal-Policy-Guidance/Downloads/ SMD-14-001.pdf.

[23] CMS, 2014 SSI and Spousal Impoverishment Standards, http://www.medicaid.gov/Medicaid-CHIP-ProgramInformation/By-Topics/Eligibility/Downloads/Spousal-Impoverishment-2014.pdf. In determining the value of home equity, states follow SSI program rules. With respect to guidance on SSI loan policy, see SSR 92-8p: Policy Interpretation Ruling Title XVI: SSI Loan Policy, Including its Applicability to Advances of Food and/or Shelter, http://www.socialsecurity.gov/OP_Home/rulings/ssi/03/SSR92-08-ssi-03.html.

[24] As per, Section 1924 of the SSA.

[25] In some cases, income that is jointly held may be attributable to the institutionalized spouse. For example, if a payment of non-trust income is made in the names of both the institutional spouse and the community spouse, half of the income is attributable to each spouse. If the income is paid from a trust, the income is considered available to each spouse depending on provisions of the trust. In the case where no provision is made on how trust income is divided and payment of income from the trust is made to each spouse, half of the income is deemed available to each spouse.

[26] CMS, 2014 SSI and Spousal Impoverishment Standards, http://www.medicaid.gov/Medicaid-CHIP-ProgramInformation/By-Topics/Eligibility/Downloads/Spousal-Impoverishment-2014.pdf.

[27] The minimum income threshold is increased to include an excess shelter allowance if the community spouse's cost of rent or mortgage payment, taxes, insurance, and utilities exceeds 30% of the amount of the minimum monthly maintenance needs allowance. A community spouse may retain additional income for every dependent family member who resides with the community spouse, so long as each family member's income is less than the minimum income threshold.

[28] CMS, 2014 SSI and Spousal Impoverishment Standards, http://www.medicaid.gov/Medicaid-CHIP-ProgramInformation/By-Topics/Eligibility/Downloads/Spousal-Impoverishment-2014.pdf.

[29] For the purposes of spousal impoverishment rules, Section 2404 of ACA redefines an "institutionalized individual" under Section 1924(h) of the SSA to include persons receiving home and community-based services (HCBS) for the five-year period beginning on January 1, 2014.

[30] The medically needy include individuals eligible for medical assistance under Section 1902(a)(10)(C) of the SSA. States may offer the medically needy pathway to individuals who are aged, blind, or disabled and have high medical expenses (including LTSS expenses) who deplete their income to specified levels.

[31] For a description of the various SSA waiver authorities and state plan LTSS coverage options, see CRS Report R43328, Medicaid Coverage of Long-Term Services and Supports, by Kirsten J. Colello.

[32] See Section 1917(c) of the SSA for requirements regarding the transfer of assets for less than fair market value.

[33] The Deficit Reduction Act of 2005 (DRA, P.L. 109-171) lengthened the look-back period from three years to five years for all asset transfers that occurred on or after the date of enactment (February 8, 2006).

[34] State Medicaid Directors Letter SMDL#14-001, ACA #29, Centers for Medicare & Medicaid Services, Department of Health and Human Services, February 21, 2014, http://www.medicaid.gov/Federal-Policy-Guidance/Downloads/ SMD-14-001.pdf.

[35] The services for which the penalty applies in the form of ineligible months for institutionalized individuals include nursing facility services; services provided in any institution in which the level of care is equivalent to those provided by a nursing facility; and Sections 1915(c) and (d) HCBS waiver services. For non-institutionalized individuals, states may extend asset transfer penalties to other state LTSS available under the state plan.

[36] Exceptions are made for transfers to a third-party by the applicant's spouse for the sole benefit of the spouse or transfers to a disabled or blind child for the sole benefit of the disabled or blind child. These transfers may include the establishment of a trust, such as a special needs trust or a pooled trust, for a disabled or blind child. These exceptions allow a spouse or parent of a disabled child to retain a source of financial support for another spouse or disabled child. States may waive asset transfer penalties for persons who would suffer undue hardship as a result of the penalty, according to criteria established by the HHS Secretary.

[37] State Medicaid Directors Letter SMDL#14-001, ACA #29, Centers for Medicare & Medicaid Services, Department of Health and Human Services, February 21, 2014, http://www.medicaid.gov/Federal-Policy-Guidance/Downloads/ SMD-14-001.pdf.

[38] DRA amended Section 1917(c)(1)(F) and (G) of the SSA to specify when the purchase of annuities should not be treated as a disposal of assets for less than FMV.

[39] Section 1917(e) of the SSA.

[40] State Medicaid Directors Letter SMDL #06-018, Centers for Medicaid and State Operations, Department of Health and Human Services, July 27, 2006, http://downloads.cms.gov/cmsgov/archived-downloads/SMDL/downloads/ SMD072706b.pdf.

[41] Section 1917(g) of the SSA.

[42] Section 3258.9 of the State Medicaid Manual, http://www.cms.gov/Regulations-and-Guidance/Guidance/Manuals/ Paper-Based-Manuals-Items/CMS021927.html.

[43] The DRA amended Section 1917(c)(1)(J) of the SSA to specify the treatment of life estates for the purposes of Medicaid asset transfer rules.

[44] Section 1917(c)(1)(I) of the SSA.

[45] Section 1917(d) of the SSA. Exemptions to asset transfer rules apply to trusts that contain the assets of a disabled individual under age 65, an income-only trust that is applied to the cost of the beneficiary's Medicaid care and for which the state is the beneficiary, and pooled trusts for disabled persons.

[46] Section 1902(q) of the SSA.

[47] Section 1915(c) of the SSA.

[48] 42 CFR 435.735.

[49] CRS Report R41899, Medicaid Eligibility for Persons Age 65+ and Individuals with Disabilities: 2009 State Profiles, by Kirsten J. Colello and Scott R. Talaga.

[50] State Medicaid Directors Letter SMDL#14-001, ACA #29, Centers for Medicare & Medicaid Services, Department of Health and Human Services, February 21, 2014, p. 6, http://www.medicaid.gov/Federal-Policy-Guidance/ Downloads/SMD-14-001.pdf.

[51] Section 1917(b) of the SSA describes estate recovery provisions.

[52] Annuities are exempt from the definition of estate if issued by a financial institution or other business that sells annuities as part of its regular business.

[53] A person's legal title or interest includes assets conveyed to a survivor, heir, or through the assignment of joint tenancy, tenancy in common, survivorship, life estate, living trust, or other arrangements.

[54] Section 1917(a) of the SSA and Section 3810.F of the State Medicaid Manual describe circumstances in which a lien may be imposed on the property of certain beneficiaries, http://www.cms.gov/Regulations-and-Guidance/Guidance/ Manuals/Paper-Based-Manuals-Items/CMS021927.html.

[55] State Medicaid Directors Letter SMDL#14-001, ACA #29, Centers for Medicare & Medicaid Services, Department of Health and Human Services, February 21, 2014, p. 6, http://www.medicaid.gov/Federal-Policy-Guidance/ Downloads/SMD-14-001.pdf.

[56] Section 3810.C of the State Medicaid Manual, http://www.cms.gov/Regulations-and-Guidance/Guidance/Manuals/ Paper-Based-Manuals-Items/CMS021927.html.

[57] Section 3810.E of the State Medicaid Manual, http://www.cms.gov/Regulations-and-Guidance/Guidance/Manuals/ Paper-Based-Manuals-Items/CMS021927.html.

[58] DRA expanded exemptions from estate recovery for those who received benefits under the Medicaid Long-Term Care Insurance Partnership Program as per Section 1917(b)(1)(C) of the SSA. As such, a private LTCI policy under the Partnership program provides a predetermined amount of assets that are disregarded, for the purposes of determining Medicaid eligibility, in the event that the lifetime benefit of the insurance plan is depleted. For example, an individual who had a dollar-for-dollar Partnership policy whose lifetime benefit is $100,000 would, upon exhausting the benefit, have $100,000 in resources exempt from Medicaid resource limits and estate recovery upon applying for Medicaid LTSS. Some Partnership policies in the original partnership states of Indiana and New York have offered policies that have total asset protection. Such policies disregard all assets of any value for the purposes of Medicaid eligibility and exempt all assets from estate recovery.

[59] State Medicaid Directors Letter SMDL#14-001, ACA #29, Centers for Medicare & Medicaid Services, Department of Health and Human Services, February 21, 2014, p. 6, http://www.medicaid.gov/Federal-Policy-Guidance/ Downloads/SMD-14-001.pdf.

In: Medicaid and Long-Term Care Assistance ISBN: 978-1-63463-328-4
Editor: Corynn D. Ford

Chapter 2

MEDICAID: FINANCIAL CHARACTERISTICS OF APPROVED APPLICANTS AND METHODS USED TO REDUCE ASSETS TO QUALIFY FOR NURSING HOME COVERAGE*

United States Government Accountability Office

WHY GAO DID THIS STUDY

Medicaid paid for nearly one-third of the nation's $158 billion in nursing home expenditures in 2012. To be financially eligible for Medicaid, individuals cannot have assets above certain limits. Not all assets are countable in determining Medicaid eligibility; federal law discourages individuals from reducing their countable assets, for example by transferring them to family members, to qualify for Medicaid. Although Congress has acted multiple times to address financial eligibility requirements for Medicaid coverage of nursing home care, methods exist through which individuals, sometimes with the help of attorneys, can reduce their assets and qualify for Medicaid.

GAO was asked for information on the extent to which individuals may be using available methods to qualify for Medicaid coverage. GAO (1) examined

---

* This is an edited, reformatted and augmented version of a United States Government Accountability Office publication, No. GAO-14-473, dated May 2014.

financial characteristics of applicants approved for Medicaid nursing home coverage in selected states;

(2) identified methods used to reduce countable assets to qualify for Medicaid; and (3) identified information eligibility workers consider the most useful in assessing applicants' financial eligibility. GAO analyzed a random, but nongeneralizeable, sample of Medicaid nursing home applications in two counties in each of three states (Florida, New York, and South Carolina), selected based on several factors including states' asset verification efforts and demographics. GAO also interviewed officials from the Centers for Medicare & Medicaid Services, state Medicaid officials, county-based Medicaid eligibility workers, and attorneys.

What GAO Found

GAO's review of 294 approved Medicaid nursing home applications in three states showed that 41 percent of applicants had total resources—both countable and not countable as part of financial eligibility determination—of $2,500 or less and 14 percent had over $100,000 in total resources.

Nearly 75 percent of applicants owned some noncountable resources, such as burial contracts; the median amount of noncountable resources was $12,530.

GAO identified four main methods used by applicants to reduce their countable assets—income or resources—and qualify for Medicaid coverage:

1) spending countable resources on goods and services that are not countable towards financial eligibility, such as prepaid funeral arrangements;
2) converting countable resources into noncountable resources that generate an income stream for the applicant, such as an annuity or promissory note;
3) giving away countable assets as a gift to another individual—such gifts could lead to a penalty period that delays Medicaid nursing home coverage; and
4) for married applicants, increasing the amount of assets a spouse remaining in the community can retain, such as through the purchase of an annuity.

Eligibility workers GAO spoke with identified bank statements as the most useful source of information for assessing financial eligibility. They explained that bank statements could lead to the identification of unreported assets, such as life insurance policies, or show patterns of withdrawals that prompt further inquiry.

The Department of Health and Human Services provided technical comments on a draft of this report, which GAO incorporated as appropriate.

ABBREVIATIONS

AVS	asset verification system
CMS	Centers for Medicare & Medicaid Services
DRA	Deficit Reduction Act of 2005
FMV	fair market value
HHS	Department of Health and Human Services
SSI	Supplemental Security Income

* * *

May 22, 2014

The Honorable Tom Coburn, M.D.
Ranking Member
Committee on Homeland Security and Governmental Affairs
United States Senate

The Honorable Richard Burr
Ranking Member
Subcommittee on Primary Health and Aging
Committee on Health, Education,
Labor, and Pensions United States Senate

The Honorable Darrell Issa
Chairman
Committee on Oversight and Government Reform
House of Representatives

The Honorable Trey Gowdy
House of Representatives

Long-term care, particularly nursing home care, can be costly; in 2012, the estimated average annual cost for an individual to receive care in a nursing home was over $85,000.[1] In that same year, nursing home expenditures in the United States amounted to $158 billion, more than half of the nation's total spending for long-term care services. Medicaid— a joint federal-state health care financing program covering certain categories of low-income individuals—is the largest payer of long-term care services and accounted for 32 percent of nursing home expenditures in 2012. As the number of elderly Americans continues to grow and more individuals are likely to need long-term care, Medicaid spending for nursing home care is projected to increase, placing additional burden on already strained federal and state resources.

Medicaid offers health care coverage, including coverage for long-term care services, to individuals whose assets—both income and resources— are insufficient to meet the costs of necessary medical services.[2] Individuals applying for Medicaid coverage for long-term care must meet certain financial and functional eligibility criteria.[3] To meet the financial eligibility criteria, individuals must have assets that fall below established standards, which vary by state, but are within standards set by the federal government. Not all assets are countable in determining financial eligibility for Medicaid. For example, states generally exclude—within specified limits—the value of an individual's primary residence, car, and prepaid burial arrangements. Additionally, federal law includes provisions to discourage individuals from reducing their countable assets—for example, by transferring them to family members—in order to establish financial eligibility for Medicaid coverage. Specifically, those who transfer assets for less than fair market value (FMV) during a specified "look-back" period—a period of time before applying for Medicaid in which an individual's or couple's assets are reviewed—may be deemed ineligible for Medicaid coverage for long-term care for a period of time called the penalty period.

As the day-to-day administrators of the Medicaid program, states are responsible for assessing applicants' financial eligibility for Medicaid coverage for long-term care; that is, determining whether an applicant's countable income and resources are below the state-established standards, and whether an applicant transferred assets for less than FMV during the look-back period. The processing of Medicaid applications is generally performed by local or county-based eligibility workers. Our previous work found that, to determine eligibility, states generally required applicants to submit applications and provide documentation of certain assets. States varied, however, in the amount of documentation required from applicants, the information they obtained from third parties to verify the accuracy of applicants' reported assets,[4] and in the proportion of applicants whom they identified as having transferred assets for less than FMV during the look-back period.[5] Some of the variation we found raised questions about whether states had sufficient information about applicants' assets to implement federal requirements. Additionally, our previous work identified methods individuals used to reduce assets to qualify for Medicaid coverage of long-term care that would not, or may not, result in a penalty period, as they would not be considered a transfer for less than FMV.[6]

Congress has acted on multiple occasions to address financial eligibility requirements for Medicaid coverage for long-term care. Most recently, the Deficit Reduction Act of 2005 (DRA), enacted in February 2006, amended some existing provisions regarding asset transfers and introduced new requirements related to financial eligibility for Medicaid coverage for long-term care.[7] For example, the DRA extended the look-back period from 36 months to 60 months for transfers occurring on or after its enactment, changed the calculation and timing of the penalty period for those transfers, and introduced new requirements for how certain types of assets—such as an individual's primary residence and an annuity— should be considered when determining Medicaid eligibility. Nevertheless, methods exist through which applicants, sometimes with the assistance of attorneys or financial planners, can reduce their assets in a manner consistent with existing law to qualify for Medicaid coverage.

Given our past work related to states' Medicaid financial eligibility determination processes, you asked us to provide information on the extent to which individuals may be using available methods to become eligible for Medicaid coverage for long-term care. In this report, we (1) examine the financial characteristics of applicants approved for Medicaid nursing home coverage in selected states; (2) identify the methods used to reduce countable assets to qualify for Medicaid coverage for nursing home care; and (3) identify the information eligibility workers considered the most useful for identifying and verifying applicants' financial eligibility.

To examine the financial characteristics of applicants approved for Medicaid nursing home coverage in selected states, we reviewed a random sample of Medicaid nursing home application files in selected counties in three states. To select the states, we determined the extent to which all states took one or more of three actions to verify applicants' reported assets using results from a 2011 GAO web-based survey of Medicaid officials from each of the 50 states and the District of Columbia.[8] On the basis of this assessment, we ranked the states on the extent to which they reported taking these actions and placed them into three groups (low, medium, and high) using naturally occurring breaks in the data. We determined whether they could provide us with needed data in order to select a sample of application files from counties within the states. We then selected 3 states—1 from the low group (Florida) and 2 from the high group (South Carolina and New York). Within each state, we selected two counties that, relative to other counties in the state, had a large number of elderly individuals (aged 65 and older), high median income of elderly households, and a high number of Medicaid nursing home applications. In total, we reviewed 350 Medicaid application files, 294 of which were approved, including those that were approved and incurred a penalty period.[9] (See app. I for information about the applications reviewed.) From the 294 approved application files, we collected and analyzed data on applicants' assets (both income and resources), whether the resources were countable toward Medicaid eligibility, and whether applicants were found to have transferred assets for less than FMV. Our analysis was limited to information included in the application files, which states used to make their eligibility determinations. We did not independently verify the accuracy of this information. However, we examined the data we collected for obvious errors and tested the data; based on this, we determined that the data were sufficiently reliable for the purposes of this report. The data from the 294 approved application files cannot be generalized to other approved applicants.

To identify the methods used to reduce countable assets to qualify for Medicaid coverage for nursing home care, we reviewed applicable federal laws and guidance, and spoke with officials from the Centers for Medicare & Medicaid Services (CMS), the agency within the Department of Health and Human Services (HHS) that oversees the Medicaid program. We interviewed nine attorneys recommended to us by the Director of the American Bar Association's Commission on Law and Aging and conducted undercover calls with representatives from 17 law offices whose websites indicated that they provided assistance to elderly individuals seeking Medicaid coverage for long-term care. We also interviewed state Medicaid officials from 12 states, and Medicaid eligibility workers from two counties in 6 of these 12 states, selected in part based on information collected from our interviews with attorneys, undercover calls with representatives from law offices, information from background literature, and demographic data on the population aged 65 and older. We supplemented this information with data collected from our review of Medicaid nursing home application files.

To identify the information eligibility workers considered the most useful for identifying and verifying applicants' financial eligibility, we used information from our interviews with county eligibility workers in two counties in each of the six states. (See app. II for more information about our scope and methodology.)

We conducted this performance audit from September 2012 to May 2014 in accordance with generally accepted government auditing standards. Those standards require that we plan and perform the audit to obtain sufficient, appropriate evidence to provide a reasonable basis for our findings and conclusions based on our audit objectives. We believe that the evidence obtained provides a reasonable basis for our findings and conclusions based on our audit objectives. We conducted our related investigative work in accordance with investigation standards prescribed by the Council of the Inspectors General on Integrity and Efficiency.

BACKGROUND

To qualify for Medicaid coverage for long-term care, including nursing home care, individuals must be within certain eligibility categories—such as those who are aged or disabled—and meet functional and financial eligibility criteria. The financial eligibility standards differ based on whether an individual is married or single. Federal law also limits Medicaid payments for long-term care for individuals who have transferred assets for less than FMV during a specified time period. States are responsible for assessing applicants' financial eligibility for Medicaid.

Financial Eligibility for Medicaid Coverage for Long-Term Care

Common ways individuals become financially eligible for Medicaid coverage of long-term care, including nursing home care, are provided below.

- Supplemental Security Income (SSI). Individuals who participate in SSI, a program that provides cash assistance to aged, blind, or disabled individuals with limited income and resources, are generally eligible for Medicaid.[10]
- Medically needy. Individuals who incur high medical costs may be able to "spend down" their income below the state-determined income

eligibility limit for Medicaid. Such individuals are referred to as "medically needy." In 2012, 32 states and the District of Columbia had a medically needy option, although not all extended this option to those who needed nursing home care.[11]

- Special income level for residents of a nursing home or institution. Individuals can qualify for Medicaid if they reside in nursing facilities or other institutions in states that have elected to establish a special income level under which individuals with incomes up to 300 percent of the SSI benefit (300 percent of the benefit was $2,163 per month in 2014) are eligible for Medicaid. In 2012, 43 states and the District of Columbia had elected this option.[12]

Some states also allow applicants to place income in excess of the special income level into a qualified income trust and receive Medicaid coverage for their care.[13] This type of trust, also known as a Miller trust, is available in states that offer the special income level option but do not also offer the medically needy option for nursing home care.[14]

The Medicaid program generally bases its characterization of assets—income and resources—for individuals who are 65 years or older or have disabilities on that used by SSI.

- Income is anything received during a calendar month, paid either in cash or in-kind, that is used or could be used to meet food or shelter needs.
- Resources are cash or real or personal property that are owned that can be converted to cash and be used for food or shelter. (See table 1 for examples of different types of assets.)

In establishing policy for determining financial eligibility for Medicaid coverage for long-term care, including nursing home care, states can decide, within federal standards, which assets are countable. For example, states may disregard certain types or amounts of income, and may elect not to count certain resources toward financial eligibility.

- Although the resources that are considered not countable varies by state, for the purposes of determining Medicaid eligibility for long-term care, they generally include an individual's primary residence (typically if the individual expresses the intent to return home), an automobile, household goods and personal effects, burial spaces, burial arrangements up to a certain value, and certain types of life insurance.

- While an individual's primary residence is generally not a countable resource for determining Medicaid eligibility, federal law specifies that an individual with substantial equity interest in his or her home is to be excluded from eligibility for Medicaid payment for long-term care; the amount of allowable equity interest is established by each state within federal guidelines. For 2014, these guidelines specified that state established allowable equity interest amounts could range from $543,000 to $814,000.[15]

Table 1. Types of Assets and Examples

Type of asset	Examples
Income	• Money earned from work • Money generated from resources, such as interest, dividends, and annuity payments[a] • Money received from other sources, such as Social Security, worker's compensation, and unemployment benefits
Resources	• Cash • Financial and investment resources, such as bank accounts, stocks,and bonds • Trusts[b] • Annuities • Real property • Vehicles, such as automobiles and boats • Life insurance • Promissory notes[c]

Source: GAO analysis of Supplemental Security Income policy.

[a]Some resources produce income. For example, an annuity is a financial instrument that provides a fixed income over a defined period of time in return for an initial payment of principal. The principal of the annuity is considered a resource, while the payments it generates are considered income.

[b]A trust is an arrangement in which a grantor transfers property to a trustee with the intention that it be held, managed, or administered by the trustee for the benefit of the grantor or certain designated individuals.

[c]A promissory note is a written, unconditional agreement, usually given in return for goods, money loaned, or services rendered, whereby one party promises to pay a certain sum of money at a specified time (or on demand) to another party.

Table 2. Income and Resource Standards for Selected Ways of Becoming Eligible for Medicaid Coverage, as of 2014

Ways of becoming eligible for Medicaid	Income standard	Resource standard
Mandatory coverage		
Supplemental Security Income (SSI)[a]	Less than $721 per month for an individual and less than $1,082 per month for a couple	Countable resources of less than $2,000 for anindividual, and less than $3,000 for a couple
State-elected coverage (optional)		
Medically needy	State-set income standard; individuals may "spend down" to eligibility by deducting incurred medical expenses from income	State-set resource standard usually no lower than countable resources of less than $2,000 for an individual or $3,000 for a couple
Special income level for residents of a nursing facility or institution	State-set income standard no higher than 300 percent of the SSI standard ($2,163 per month) for an individual[b]	Same as SSI

Sources: GAO analysis of Medicaid eligibility requirements.

[a]Not all SSI recipients automatically qualify for Medicaid. Under Section 1902(f) of the Social Security Act, a state may use more restrictive Medicaid eligibility standards than SSI's standards, provided the standards are no more restrictive than those the state had in place as of January 1, 1972. As of March 2013, 11 states had opted to use these standards. These states are often referred to as 209(b) states because the origin of this provision was § 209(b) of the Social Security Amendments of 1972, Pub. L. No. 92-603, 86 Stat. 1329, 1381.

[b]Some states also allow applicants to place income in excess of the special income level into a qualified income trust and receive Medicaid coverage for their care. This type of trust, also known as a Miller trust, is available in states that offer the special income level option but do not also offer the medically needy option for nursing home care.

In most states, to be financially eligible for Medicaid coverage for long-term care, including nursing home care, individuals must have $2,000 or less in countable resources ($3,000 for a married couple). However, specific income and resource standards vary depending on the way an individual becomes eligible for Medicaid. (See table 2.) Eligible individuals generally must contribute a portion of their income toward the costs of nursing home care but are allowed to retain a small personal needs allowance, which varies by state but must be at least $30 per month, to pay for the individual's clothing and other personal needs.

Spousal Impoverishment Protections

Federal law requires states to use specific minimum and maximum income and resource standards in determining Medicaid eligibility for married applicants when one spouse is in an institution (referred to as the institutionalized spouse), such as a nursing home, and the other remains in the community (referred to as the community spouse).[16] These provisions enable the institutionalized spouse to become eligible for Medicaid, while leaving the community spouse with sufficient assets to avoid impoverishment.

- **Resources**. The resources of both the institutionalized spouse and the community spouse are considered when determining initial financial eligibility for Medicaid coverage for nursing home care. The community spouse may retain an amount equal to one-half of the couple's combined countable resources, up to the state-specified maximum resource level. States' maximum resource levels cannot exceed the maximum federal standard, which was $117,240 for 2014.[17] The amount that the community spouse is allowed to retain is generally referred to as the community spouse resource allowance.[18]
- **Income**. A community spouse's income is not considered when determining financial eligibility for Medicaid coverage for nursing home care; the community spouse is allowed to retain all of his or her own income. States establish, within federal standards, a minimum amount of income—a minimum needs allowance—that a community spouse is entitled to retain.[19] If the community spouse's income is less than the minimum needs allowance, then income from the institutionalized spouse can be transferred to the community spouse to make up the difference.[20] As of January 1, 2014, federal standards specified that most states' minimum needs allowance can be no lower than $1,938.75, and no higher than $2,931.00 per month.[21]

Transfers of Assets

Federal law limits Medicaid payment for long-term care services, including nursing home care, for individuals who divest themselves of—or "transfer"—their assets for less than FMV within a specified time period.[22] As a result, when an individual applies for Medicaid coverage for longterm care, states conduct a review, or "look-back," to determine whether the applicant (or his or her spouse, if married) transferred assets to another person or party. Per the DRA, the look-back period for transfers made on or after February 8, 2006, is 60 months; prior to the DRA, the look-back period was generally 36 months. If the state determines that an applicant transferred an asset for less than FMV during the look-back period, the individual may be ineligible for Medicaid coverage for longterm care for a period of time, called the penalty period.[23]

The penalty period generally begins on the later of (1) the first day of a month during or after an individual transfers assets for less than FMV, or (2) the date on which the individual would otherwise be eligible to receive coverage for services were it not for the penalty period.

Federal law exempts certain transfers made during the look-back period from the penalty provisions.

Exemptions include certain transfers of assets to a spouse or a disabled child, among other things.[24] A transfer does not result in a penalty period if the individual can demonstrate to the state that the transfer was made exclusively for purposes other than qualifying for Medicaid.[25] Additionally, a penalty would not be applied if the state determined that application of the penalty would result in an undue hardship; that is, it would deprive the individual of (1) medical care such that the individual's health or life would be endangered, or (2) food, clothing, shelter, or other necessities for life.

The DRA also specified circumstances under which the purchase of certain assets—such as an annuity, promissory note, or loan—is considered a transfer for less than FMV for purposes of determining Medicaid eligibility. (See table 3 for a summary of these selected DRA provisions.) Most, but not all, of these provisions became applicable on the date of the DRA's enactment, February 8, 2006.

Table 3. Summary of Selected Provisions Regarding Transfers of Assets in the Deficit Reduction Act of 2005 (DRA)

DRA provision	Description
Annuities[a]	• States are required to treat the purchase of an annuity as a transfer for less than fair market value (FMV) unless the annuity names the state as either (1) the remainder beneficiary in the first position for at least the total amount of Medicaid expenditures paid on behalf of the annuitant, or (2) a remainder beneficiary in the second position after the community spouse, orminor or disabled child (or in the first position if any of those individuals transfer the remainder of the annuity for less than FMV). • Annuities purchased by or on the behalf of an individual who applied for Medicaid coverage forlong-term care shall be treated as a transfer of assets for less than FMV unless the annuity is irrevocable, nonassignable, actuarially sound, and provides for payments in equal amounts during the term of the annuity, with no deferral and no balloon payments. • Annuities purchased by or on the behalf of an individual who applied for Medicaid coverage forlong-term care services that are defined as individual retirement accounts under federal tax code, or purchased with the proceeds of certain retirement accounts and meet certain federal tax code requirements are not considered transfers for less than FMV.
Life estates	States are required to consider a purchase of a life estate interest in another person's home as a transfer of assets for less than FMV unless the purchaser lived in the home for at least 1 year after the date of purchase.
Promissory notes and loans	States are required to consider funds used to purchase a promissory note, loan, or mortgage as a transfer of assets for less than FMV unless the repayment terms are actuarially sound, provide for payments to be made in equal amounts during the term of the loan with no deferral or balloon payments, and prohibit the cancellation of the balance upon the death of the lender.

Source: GAO analysis of the DRA.

[a]The DRA also specified that applications for Medicaid coverage for long-term care shall: (1) describe any interest an applicant or community spouse may have in an annuity, regardless of whether the annuity is irrevocable or treated as an asset; and (2) include a statement that the state becomes a remainder beneficiary of an annuity purchased on or after enactment by virtue of the applicant's receipt of Medicaid assistance for long-term care.

States' Determination of Applicants' Financial Eligibility

To assess applicants' financial eligibility for Medicaid coverage for long-term care, including nursing home care, and to determine whether they transferred assets for less than FMV, states generally require applicants to submit applications and to provide documentation of certain assets reported on the applications.

Our prior work has shown that states varied in the amount of documentation required from applicants; for example, 17 states required all applicants to provide 60 months of documentation of financial and investment resources, while 27 states required applicants to provide just the current month's documentation.

We also previously found that all state Medicaid programs obtained some amount of asset information from third parties, such as financial institutions or other government agencies, such as the Social Security Administration.[26] Such information helps states verify the accuracy of applicants' reported assets, and to determine if applicants have assets they failed to report or transferred for less than FMV during thc look-back period. The processing of Medicaid applications—including the collection of documentation and information from applicants and third parties—is generally performed by local or county-based eligibility workers.

Files Reviewed Showed 41 Percent of Approved Applicants Had Total Resources at or below $2,500, and 5 Percent Transferred Assets

Forty-one percent of the 294 approved applicants whose Medicaid nursing home application files we reviewed had total resources—both countable and not countable resources—of $2,500 or less; and nearly 75 percent of the approved applicants owned at least some resources that were not countable in their financial eligibility determination. Almost two-thirds of approved applicants had annual gross incomes of $20,000 or less, and 5 percent were found to have transferred assets for less than FMV.

Forty-One Percent of Approved Applicants Reviewed Had Total Resources of $2,500 or Less; Nearly Three-Quarters Had Some Resources Not Countable for Eligibility Determination

Of the 294 approved Medicaid nursing home applicants whose files we reviewed in selected counties in three states, 41 percent—121 applicants—had total resources of $2,500 or less. Total resources included both resources that were countable and those that were not countable as part of applicants' Medicaid financial eligibility determination and, for married applicants, resources of both the applicant and the spouse. Another 44 percent of approved applicants—129 applicants— had between $2,501 and $100,000 in total resources, and 14 percent of approved applicants—42 applicants—had over $100,000 in total resources.[27] Median total resources for all approved applicants was $7,660,[28] which was less than the median net worth of elderly households in the United States.[29] Married applicants, who made up 24 percent of the approved applicants, had higher median resources ($70,137) than single applicants ($3,034).[30] (See fig. 1.)

Approved applicants most commonly owned the following types of resources: financial and investment resources (95 percent), burial contracts and prepaid funeral arrangements (39 percent), life insurance policies (34 percent), their primary residence (31 percent), and vehicles (26 percent). With the exception of the applicant's primary residence, the median value of these more commonly owned resources was less than that of other resources—namely annuities, life estates, promissory notes, or trusts—that were less commonly owned. (See table 4.)

Certain types of resources, such as prepaid burial arrangements, are generally not countable for purposes of determining Medicaid eligibility. Of the approved applicants whose files we reviewed, 74 percent (218 of 294) owned at least some resources that were not countable as part of their financial eligibility determination, though the amount of noncountable resources owned varied. Files for 195 of these 218 applicants contained information on the value of at least one noncountable resource owned.[31] Among these 195 applicants, 55 percent (108 applicants) had $20,000 or less in noncountable resources, 27 percent (53 applicants) had noncountable resources between $20,001 and $100,000, and 17 percent (34 applicants) had greater than $100,000 in resources that were not countable toward eligibility. The median value of noncountable resources was $12,530.[32]

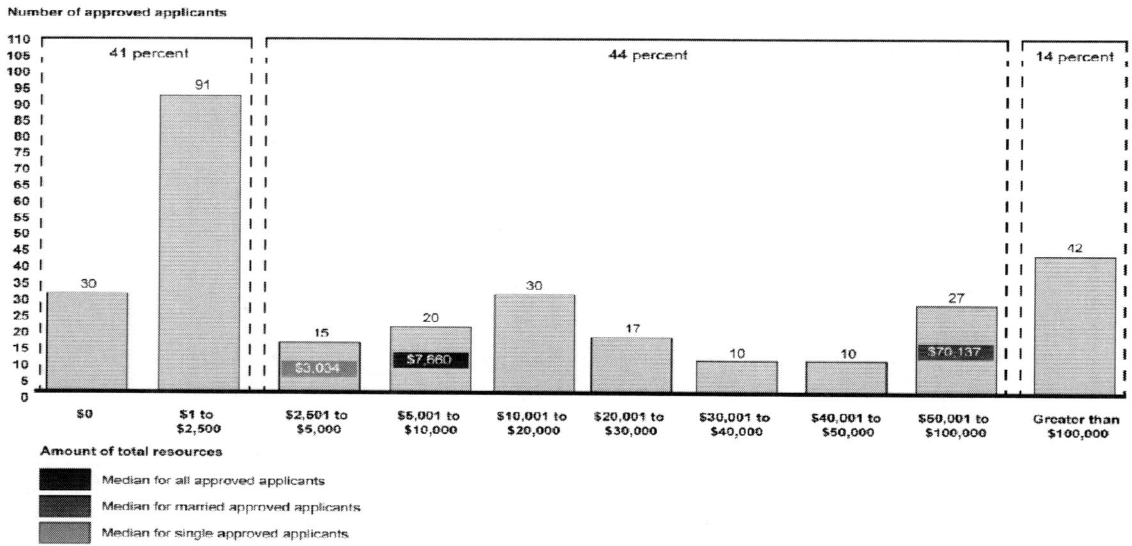

Notes: Data for four counties were from applications submitted during state fiscal year 2012, while data for two counties were from applications submitted between July 1, 2012, and December 31, 2012.

Consistent with how Medicaid eligibility is determined for coverage of nursing home care, our analysis of total resources for married applicants includes those of both the spouse and the applicant.

For 2 of the 294 approved applicants who owned at least one resource, there was no information available on the value of any of their resources. As such, the percentages shown do not add to 100. Files for the remaining applicants included information on the value of at least one resource; all known values were summed to determine the total resources per applicant. However, if an applicant's file did not contain a value for every resource the applicant owned, then the amount of their total resources may be underestimated.

Figure 1. Distribution of Approved Applicants in Selected Counties in Three States by Amount of Total Resources (n=294).

Table 4. Number of Approved Applicants in Selected Counties in Three States that Owned Resources, and the Value of Resources Owned, by Type of Resource

Resource	Number (percent) of approved applicants who owned resource	Number of applicants for whom the value of a resource owned was known	Median value of resource
Financial and investment[b]	278 (95%)	277	$1,200
Burial contracts and prepaid funeral arrangements	114 (39%)	95	$9,311
Life insurance	101 (34%)	86	$2,422
Primary residence	91 (31%)	66	$68,350
Vehicle	77 (26%)	51	$3,110
Life estate	10 (3%)	4	$71,550
Real property other than primary residence	10 (3%)	10	$47,300
Trust	9 (3%)	4	$82,000
Promissory note or loan	5 (2%)	5	$116,500
Annuity	3 (1%)	2	$44,261
Other resources c	6 (2%)	3	$1,361

Source: GAO analysis of Medicaid application data.

Notes: Data for four counties were from applications submitted during state fiscal year 2012, while data for two counties were from applications submitted between July 1, 2012, and December 31, 2012.

Consistent with how Medicaid eligibility is determined for coverage of nursing home care, resources for married applicants include those of both the spouse and the applicant.

[a]The value of a resource was considered to be known if the applicant's file included information on the value for at least one of that type of resource. For example, if an applicant had two bank accounts, the value of financial and investment resources was considered to be known if the applicant's file included information on the value of at least one of the accounts. Missing values may have affected the median values of each type of resource.

[b]Financial and investment resources includes such items as checking or savings bank accounts, stocks, bonds, and retirement accounts.

[c]Other resources include such items as cash, livestock, and unspecified property in safety deposit boxes or storage units.

Approved applicants who were married had a greater median value of noncountable resources ($60,651) than single applicants ($9,931), which could be due, in part, to Medicaid eligibility rules that include provisions intended to protect the community spouse from impoverishment.[33] (See fig. 2.)

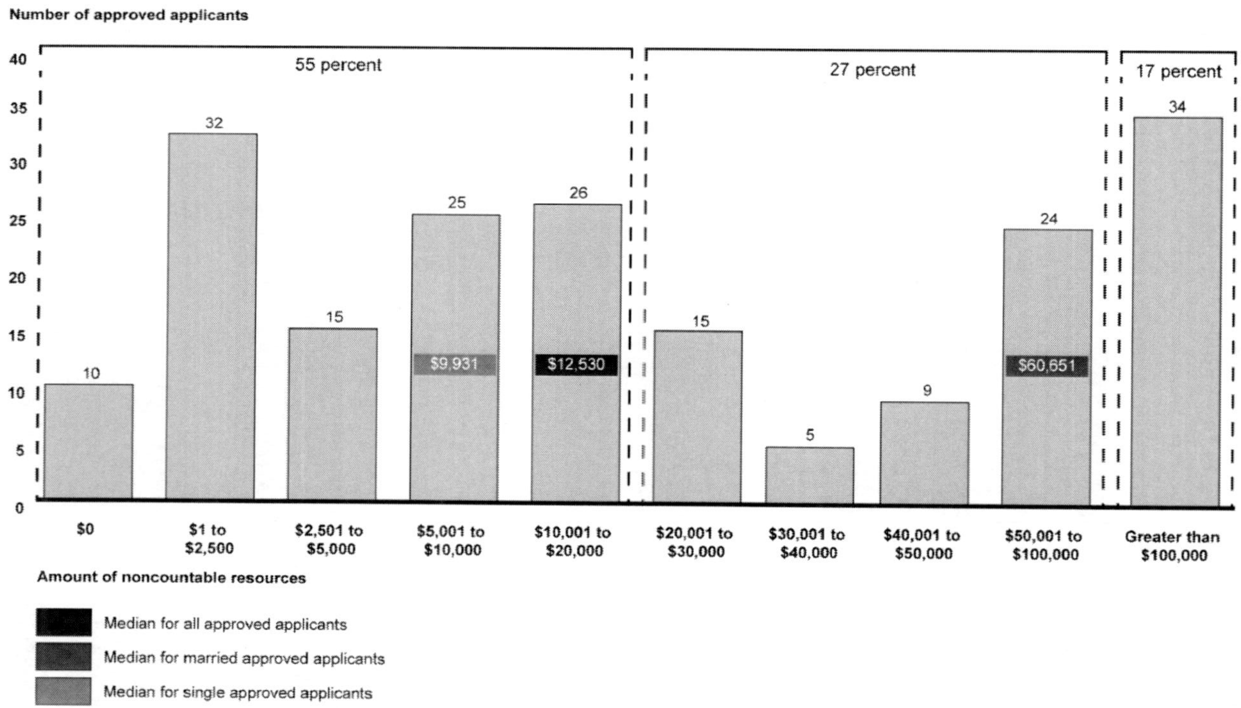

Source: GAO analysis of Medicaid application data.

Notes: Data for four counties were from applications submitted during state fiscal year 2012, while data for two counties were from applications submitted between July 1, 2012, and December 31, 2012.

Within federal standards, states may elect not to count certain resources toward financial eligibility. Thus, the amount of noncountable resources reflects the value of the applicant's resources that the state elected not to count during eligibility determination. Consistent with how Medicaid eligibility is determined for coverage of nursing home care, noncountable resources for married applicants include those of both the spouse and the applicant.

Of the 294 approved applicants whose files we reviewed, 218 owned at least one noncountable resource. For 23 of these 218 approved applicants, there was no information available on the value of their noncountable resources. Files for the remaining 195 applicants included information on the value of at least one noncountable resource; all known values were summed to determine the amount of noncountable resources per applicant. However, if an applicant's file did not contain a value for every noncountable resource the applicant owned, then the amount of their noncountable resources may be underestimated.

Percentages shown do not add to 100 due to rounding.

Figure 2. Distribution of Approved Applicants in Selected Counties in Three States by Amount of Noncountable Resources (n=195).

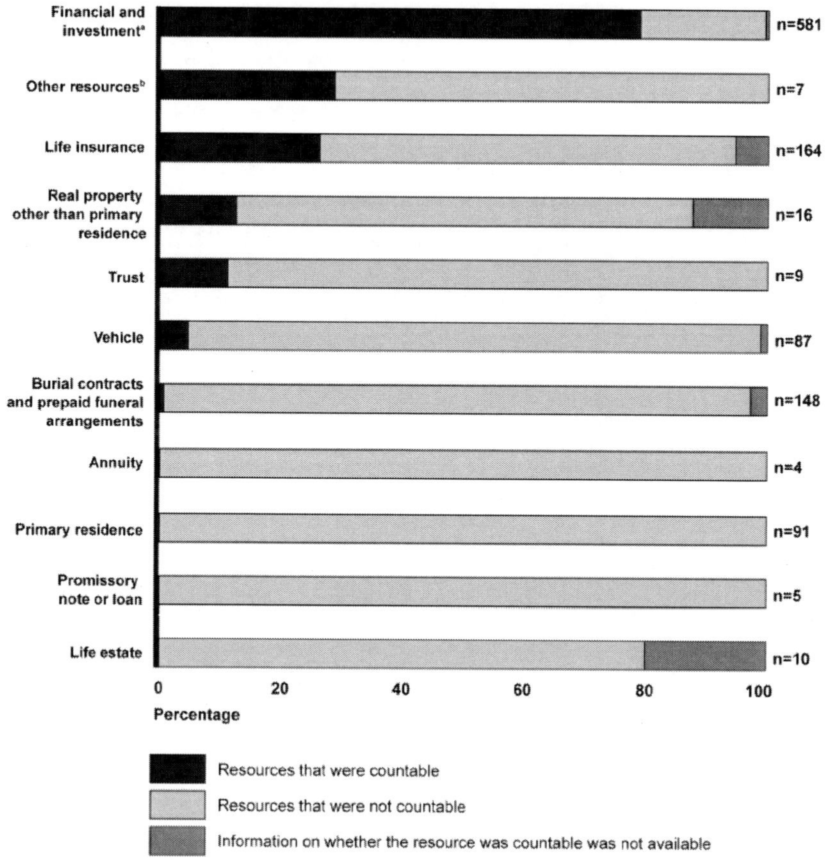

Notes: Data for four counties were from applications submitted during state fiscal year 2012, while data for two counties were from applications submitted between July 1, 2012, and December 31, 2012.

[a]Financial and investment resources includes such items as checking or savings bank accounts, stocks, bonds, and retirement accounts.

[b]Other resources include such items as cash, livestock, and unspecified property in safety deposit boxes or storage units.

Figure 3. Proportion of Resources that Were Countable as Part of Applicants' Financial Eligibility Among Approved Applicants in Selected Counties in Three States, by Type of Resource.

The extent to which the types of resources applicants owned were countable toward applicants' eligibility varied. While 79 percent of the financial and investment resources owned by approved applicants were countable, the majority of vehicles, and burial contracts and prepaid funeral arrangements were not countable as part of eligibility determination. Additionally, none of the applicants' annuities, promissory notes, or primary residences were countable. (See fig. 3.) Although an applicant's primary residence is typically not a countable resource, an applicant with significant equity interest in his or her home is not eligible for Medicaid payments for nursing home care.[34] For the 51 applicants for whom we were able to determine the equity interest in the home, the median home equity was $50,000, and ranged from $0 to $700,000.

Almost Two-Thirds of Approved Applicants Reviewed Had Income of $20,000 or Less

Sixty-five percent of approved applicants whose files we reviewed—192 applicants—had annual gross incomes of $20,000 or less, another 30 percent—88 applicants—had annual gross incomes between $20,001 and $50,000, and 5 percent—14 applicants—had annual gross incomes greater than $50,000.[35] The median annual gross income of approved applicants was $16,260 ($1,355 per month),[36] which was less than the median annual income of the elderly in the United States.[37] In contrast to resources, the median annual gross income of married approved applicants ($16,260) was nearly the same as that of their single counterparts ($16,284); consistent with how Medicaid eligibility is determined, applicants' income includes just that of the applicant, regardless of marital status. (See fig. 4.)

Social Security was the primary source of income for approved applicants we reviewed, comprising three-quarters of their annual income, on average. Almost all approved applicants—95 percent—received Social Security, and nearly half—45 percent—received income from a retirement account or pension. Few applicants received income from other sources, such as an annuity, trust, or promissory note.

For slightly more than half (33) of the 60 married approved applicants who had a spouse living in the community, the community spouse was allowed to retain at least some of the applicant's income to bring their monthly income up to the state's minimum needs allowance. The median value of the amount of the applicant's income that the community spouse was allowed to retain was $1,102 per month.[38]

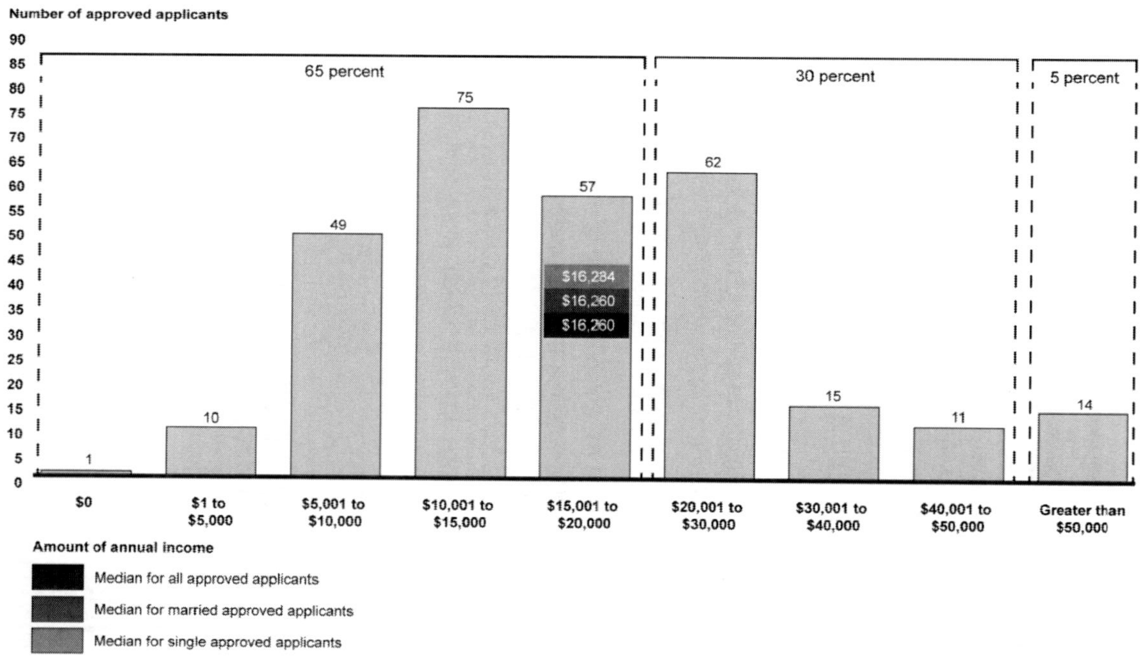

Notes: Data for four counties were from applications submitted during state fiscal year 2012, while data for two counties were from applications submitted between July 1, 2012, and December 31, 2012.

Consistent with how Medicaid eligibility is determined for coverage of nursing home care, income includes just that of the applicant, regardless of the applicant's marital status.

Figure 4. Distribution of Approved Applicants in Selected Counties in Three States by Annual Gross Income.

Files Reviewed Showed Five Percent of Approved Applicants Transferred Assets for Less Than Fair Market Value

Files for 5 percent of approved applicants reviewed—15 applicants—showed transfers of assets for less than FMV during the look-back period; such transfers are to result in the assessment of a penalty period. The median amount of assets transferred was $24,608, and the amounts ranged from $5,780 to $296,221. The majority of applicants identified as transferring assets for less than FMV—14 of the 15 applicants— transferred money. Applicants typically transferred assets to a child or grandchild (9 of the 15 applicants). Thirteen of the 15 applicants found to have transferred assets were not married. All but one of the applicants found to have transferred assets were from New York, the remaining applicant was from South Carolina.[39] Among applicants found to have transferred assets, the median length of the penalty period assessed was nearly 4 months, and the length ranged from half a month to nearly 25 months.

Applicants Used Four Main Methods to Reduce Countable Assets and Qualify for Medicaid

We identified four main methods used by applicants—or described by eligibility workers, state officials, attorneys, or other representatives from law practices—to reduce countable assets and qualify for Medicaid coverage for nursing home care. These four methods are: (1) spending countable resources on goods and services that are not countable, (2) converting countable resources into noncountable resources that generate an income stream, (3) giving away countable assets, and (4) increasing the amount of assets the community spouse retains.

Spending Countable Resources on Goods and Services That Are Not Countable Toward Financial Eligibility

One method Medicaid applicants could use to reduce assets is paying off existing debt or making certain purchases. When such purchases and payments convert a countable resource, such as money in the bank, into a good or service that is not countable toward Medicaid financial eligibility, they effectively reduce the applicants' assets. Eligibility workers mentioned possible goods that would not be countable that applicants could purchase.

- Eligibility workers in 10 of the 12 counties interviewed stated that purchasing burial contracts and prepaid funeral arrangements, which are generally noncountable resources, was a common way applicants reduced their countable assets; and eligibility workers from one state said they recommend making such purchases to applicants.
- Eligibility workers also reported that applicants spend down their countable resources on upgrades to their homes, such as a new roof or carpeting.

States may require applicants to provide documentation related to these purchases, such as construction contracts or receipts, to verify that the purchases were not made for less than FMV.

Applicants can also use countable resources to purchase services, which are not considered a resource. For example, applicants may pay for a personal service contract, also referred to as a care agreement, which is an arrangement in which an individual pays another person, often an adult child, to provide certain services—such as grocery shopping or transportation to medical appointments—over a period of time. Although personal service contracts are not considered a resource, payment for the contracts involve a transfer of resources, and thus must be assessed to determine whether the transfer was made for less than FMV. If such contracts are determined to have been made for less than FMV, then the applicant would be subject to a penalty period. According to CMS, states can establish reasonable standards for assessing whether or not a transfer using a personal service contract is made for less than FMV. Our interviews with state Medicaid officials indicate that states' standards for assessing the FMV of personal service contracts vary.

- Some states require that payments under the contract be made at the time the services are rendered; thus, these states would consider a lump sum payment made for services that had been provided sometime in the past or for services that will be provided in the future to be a transfer for less than FMV.
- In contrast, officials from one state we spoke with indicated that the state does not have standards regarding when payment must be made. Officials from this state reported seeing at least 100 applications each month containing personal service contracts.

Personal Service Contracts

The files we reviewed included a $7,055 personal service contract between an applicant and her daughter for the provision of 10 hours of care per week at a rate of $11 per hour for an estimated 1.2 years. Another applicant had a $134,316 contract with her son to provide 20 hours of services per week at a rate of $35 per hour for an estimated 3.7 years. Under both personal service contracts, the provider received one lump sum payment.

Among the Medicaid application files that we reviewed in selected states, 16 of the 294 approved applicants (5 percent) had a personal service contract—all of which were determined to be for FMV. The median value of the personal service contracts was $37,000; the value of the contracts ranged from $4,460 to $250,004.

Converting Countable Resources into Noncountable Resources That Generate an Income Stream for the Applicant

Applicants may reduce their countable resources by purchasing certain financial instruments that generate an income stream. While the income stream is likely countable, the principal of the financial instrument might not be a countable resource when determining an applicant's financial eligibility. For these purchases to be effective in helping the individual qualify for Medicaid coverage, the income generated would need to be less than the applicant's expenses, including the cost of nursing home care; otherwise the applicant would not likely be income-eligible for Medicaid coverage for nursing home care. Additionally, the principal would need to be a noncountable resource, otherwise the applicant would not likely be resource-eligible for Medicaid coverage.

Irrevocable Annuities

In certain circumstances an irrevocable annuity can be considered a countable resource. For example, according to CMS, if the annuity can be sold on the secondary market because its owner or payee may be changed (i.e., the annuity is assignable), then the annuity is a countable resource.

One instrument applicants can purchase to convert countable resources into noncountable resources with an income stream is an irrevocable and nonassignable annuity that complies with the DRA.[40] A representative from one law office that we spoke to in an undercover capacity indicated that an annuity is an option that could allow at least some resources to be left for the applicant's heirs. While the individual noted that the income generated from the annuity must be spent on nursing home care, he explained that the applicant may be able to save some money to leave to his children because the amount the applicant would have to pay toward his nursing home care would be based on the Medicaid nursing home payment rate, which is likely less than what the applicant would have otherwise had to pay privately. Medicaid officials from more than half the states for which we conducted interviews indicated that the use of annuities has increased over the past few years, and officials from one of these states indicated that this increase was a result of clearer guidelines in the DRA on annuities.

Another financial instrument applicants may be able to purchase to convert countable resources into noncountable resources with an income stream is a promissory note, under which applicants lend funds to another party, such as an adult child.[41] States are required to determine whether the funds used to purchase a promissory note were a transfer for less than FMV.[42] Additionally, according to CMS officials, if a promissory note is determined to have been purchased at FMV, states must also determine whether the principal of the note should be treated as a countable resource. Based on our interviews with state Medicaid officials, states' standards for determining whether to treat the principal of promissory notes as a countable resource vary.

- Medicaid officials from one state told us that the principal of promissory notes could be considered a countable resource if it were negotiable.
- Medicaid officials from another state said that the principal would be a countable resource if the note could be converted into cash within 20 days.

Giving Away Some or All Countable Assets

Applicants may reduce their countable assets by giving some or all of their assets as a gift to another individual, such as an adult child. Such gifts are typically treated as a transfer for less than FMV and, if given during the look-back period, would likely result in a penalty period. The length of the penalty period is calculated based on the value of the gift and the private payment rate for nursing home services in the state or locality.[43] However, our interviews identified mechanisms that either reduce the length of the penalty period after it has started or provide funds to pay for care during the penalty period. These mechanisms are referred to as "reverse half-a-loaf" because they can be used to preserve at least half of an individual's resources.[44]

A "reverse half-a-loaf" mechanism that reduces the length of the penalty period involves gifting countable assets to someone else and then, after eligibility has been determined and the penalty period begins, having a portion of the gift returned to the applicant. This option only works in states that choose to consider a partial return of transferred assets in recalculating the penalty period. According to CMS, states can choose whether or not to consider a partial return of transferred assets. In states that consider partial returns, the original length of the penalty period would be shortened in proportion to the amount of assets returned.[45]

Another "reverse half-a-loaf" mechanism involves an applicant gifting a portion of their countable resources, incurring a penalty, and converting other countable resources into an income stream for the applicant—such as through an annuity or promissory note—to pay for nursing home care during the penalty period. The amount of income generated from the annuity or promissory note would be equivalent to the shortfall between the applicant's other monthly income, such as Social Security and retirement income, and the cost of his/her nursing home care during the penalty period. A representative from one law office we spoke to in an undercover capacity suggested that the applicant could gift about 50 percent of her resources, and while serving a penalty period, the applicant would use monthly income from a promissory note plus other monthly income to pay for the nursing home care. Another representative from a law office mentioned that the larger the applicant's income, the larger the amount that the applicant can gift. This is because an applicant with higher income would need less additional income from an annuity or promissory note to cover the costs of nursing home services during the penalty period.

Thus, an applicant with higher income would need to place a smaller amount of their countable resources into an annuity or promissory note, allowing them to gift more of their countable resources even if it may result in a longer penalty period.

Reverse Half-a-Loaf

One applicant who appeared to use the "reverse half-a-loaf" mechanism gifted $62,470 to his children and was assessed a 6 month penalty period. This applicant also loaned $63,118 to one of his children in return for a promissory note that provided $10,543 in income per month during the 6 months of the applicant's penalty period.

Among the 294 approved applicants whose files we reviewed, we identified 5 applicants (2 percent) who appeared to have used one of the "reverse half-a-loaf" mechanisms; 4 of the applicants appeared to use the mechanism that involved creating an income stream through a promissory note to pay for nursing home care during the penalty period. These 4 applicants gifted between $20,150 and $227,250 worth of resources, and had penalty periods of between 2 months and 22 months.

Increasing the Amount of Assets the Community Spouse Retains

An additional method married applicants could use to reduce countable assets is to increase the amount of assets that the community spouse is able to retain. Given the federal law regarding the treatment of the community spouse's resources and provisions intended to protect married individuals, there are several different mechanisms for increasing the assets retained by the community spouse.

Spousal Refusal

Federal law permits the community spouse to retain an amount equal to one-half of the couple's combined countable resources, up to the state-specified maximum resource level. However, our work identified a mechanism that could result in a community spouse retaining more than the maximum standard in instances where the state did not exercise its right to sue the community spouse to recoup the resources due to the institutionalized spouse. Under this mechanism, an institutionalized spouse may transfer all his or her resources to the community spouse, while assigning to the state the right to bring a support proceeding against the community spouse.[46] In this way, a community spouse who refuses to make any resources available to the institutionalized spouse may be able to retain all of the couple's resources unless the state chooses to sue the community spouse for support.[47] According to information from state officials, some states take legal action to recoup funds from the community spouse in cases of spousal refusal, while other states do not.

- Medicaid officials from one state told us that they do not see many applications claiming spousal refusal, adding this is likely because the state would take legal action against the community spouse to recoup expenses.
- Officials from other states told us that, in cases of spousal refusal, they do not take action against the community spouse.

Of the 70 married approved applicants whose files we reviewed, 13 had applications that contained a claim of spousal refusal. (See table 5.) These 13 applicants resided in two states and the community spouse retained a median value of $291,888 in nonhousing resources; two of the community spouses were able to retain over $1 million in nonhousing resources.[48] Six of the 13 applicants also provided monthly income support to their community spouse.[49]

Table 5. Amount of Nonhousing Resources and Monthly Income Support Retained by the Community Spouse in Cases of Spousal Refusal, for Approved Applicants in Selected Counties in Three States

Applicant	Amount of nonhousing resources retained by the community spouse	Amount of monthly income provided by the institutionalized spouse to the community spouse
1	$13,306	$0
2	$47,214	$1,874
3	$126,627	$441
4	$146,862	$0
5	$194,912	$0
6	$212,611	$0
7	$291,888	$770
8	$352,936	$0
9	$394,189	$1,734
10	$432,860	$0
11	$452,251	$1,588
12	$1,429,209	$2,088
13	$1,585,467	$0

Source: GAO analysis of Medicaid application data.

Note: Data for four counties were from applications submitted during state fiscal year 2012, while data for two counties were from applications submitted between July 1, 2012, and December 31, 2012.

Annuities for the Community Spouse

Married applicants may reduce their countable assets by purchasing an irrevocable and nonassignable annuity that pays out income to the community spouse. Although annuities for the community spouse must be actuarially sound—that is, they must pay out during the community spouse's life expectancy—and must name the state as a remainder beneficiary, there are no other limitations on the time period in which annuities must pay out. Additionally, there is no limit on the amount of income from the annuity, as the community spouse's income is not countable as part of the institutionalized spouse's eligibility. While any portion of the income from the annuity that is not spent in the month it is received becomes a resource, a community spouse's resources are generally not assessed again after his or her spouse is initially deemed eligible, and thus would not affect the institutionalized spouse's eligibility.[50]

Annuities for the Community Spouse

State Medicaid officials, county eligibility workers, and attorneys who provided information on the value of annuities for the community spouse reported average values ranging from $50,000 to $300,000. Officials from one state reported seeing annuities for the community spouse worth more than $1 million. Medicaid officials from one state indicated that they have seen annuities that disbursed all of the payments to the community spouse shortly after the annuity was purchased, while officials from another state said that annuities can have large monthly payments for the community spouse, such as $10,000 per month.

Thus, married applicants may use countable resources to purchase an irrevocable annuity that pays potentially large amounts of income for the community spouse over a short period of time without affecting the institutionalized spouse's eligibility. A representative from one law office we spoke to in an undercover capacity suggested that the creation of an annuity can be done quickly and therefore, is a tool for last minute planning. Similar to the annuities for the applicant, Medicaid officials from several states said that the use of annuities for the community spouse has increased over the past few years. Officials from three states said that the increase may be a result of the passage of the DRA, because it clarified how annuities for the community spouse could be set up.

Court Order of Support

Married applicants may seek a court order that requires the institutionalized spouse to pay a specified monthly income or provide additional resources to support the community spouse. Such court orders could allow the community spouse to receive income or resources in excess of maximum standards. Federal law requires that a community spouse's income allowance be no less than the amount of the court order of support.[51]

One state Medicaid official that we spoke to said that applicants who use court orders will have a preeligibility asset test, or needs assessment, conducted to determine the amount of excess resources that the married couple would have to spend down before applying for Medicaid, after which they will seek a court order of resource support that allows the spouse to keep an amount of the couple's combined resources that is above the state's maximum resource allowance. Of the 70 married approved applicants whose files we reviewed, 1 applicant had a court order of spousal income support that required the institutionalized applicant to divert $5,014 of her monthly income to the community spouse, which was greater than the state's minimum needs allowance.

ELIGIBILITY WORKERS CONSIDERED BANK STATEMENTS THE MOST USEFUL SOURCE TO IDENTIFY AND VERIFY APPLICANTS' FINANCIAL ELIGIBILITY

Eligibility workers from all 12 counties in which we conducted interviews stated that bank statements were the most useful source of information for identifying and verifying applicants' financial eligibility. According to the eligibility workers we spoke with, bank statements show transactions, such as payments of life insurance premiums, the movement of lump sums of money over time, or transfers of money in and out of accounts. Presumably, these workers had access to itemized bank statements— periodic statements issued by a financial institution to its customers detailing all account activity for that period. Eligibility workers from one county said that bank statements allowed them to best understand an applicant's financial history. Additionally, bank statements can include red flags or triggers that can lead eligibility workers to ask the applicant for additional information.

- For example, eligibility workers from counties in which we conducted interviews indicated that large withdrawals or patterns of withdrawals, incomplete documentation (e.g., missing pages), or an applicant having a large number of accounts can prompt further inquiry.
- Eligibility workers also reported that reviews of bank statements could lead to the identification of unreported assets or accounts. The most commonly unreported asset those eligibility workers reported finding in bank statements were life insurance policies. Specifically, eligibility workers from 7 of the 12 counties in which we conducted interviews reported that life insurance policies are commonly not reported and may be found while reviewing itemized bank statements because the statements may show a payment for the life insurance premium. Life insurance policies that have a cash value could affect an applicant's eligibility.

Although eligibility workers indicated that bank statements are the most useful source of information on applicants' assets, we have previously found that over half of states require only a single month's documentation for financial and investment resources, such as bank accounts.[52] Having only a single month's bank statement could be sufficient to determine the current value of an applicant's account, but it may not allow eligibility workers to identify patterns of withdrawals over time which could indicate the need for additional review. All the eligibility workers we interviewed, however, said they ask for additional information if they see large withdrawals in the bank statements that were submitted. For example, eligibility workers from one county that requires only a single month of documentation said if there is questionable information in the documentation they will request that the applicant submit additional months of documentation. Additionally, we previously found that few states require applicants to provide itemized bank statements as documentation of their resources.[53] While applicants may submit itemized bank statements even if not required, without such detailed statements, eligibility workers may not be able to discover unreported assets, such as life insurance policies.

Some eligibility workers we interviewed indicated that applicants' income tax returns were also a helpful source of information to identify applicants' unreported assets. Specifically, eligibility workers from three counties (in two states) told us that that they ask applicants for a copy of their federal tax return. For example, eligibility workers from one county stated that they require applicants to provide 5 years of tax returns. These workers indicated that income tax returns include much information that workers would otherwise not be able to access, such as information about ownership of life insurance policies, stocks, or any other asset that earns dividends. In our previous work, we found that only one state requires the submission of income tax returns.[54]

In addition to bank statements and tax returns, eligibility workers also reported finding some asset-related search tools helpful in identifying and verifying applicants' assets and transfers. Workers from one county in Florida that had recently begun piloting an electronic asset verification system (AVS)[55]—a system that allows workers to contact multiple financial institutions to determine if an applicant has, or had, an account and the value of any existing accounts—noted that this new system has been useful in identifying unreported assets and transfers.[56] The state's AVS collects information from participating banks on any accounts held by an applicant for nursing home coverage in the prior 60 months. If a bank account is found, the information is populated into the state's electronic eligibility system for eligibility workers to use in evaluating applicants' financial eligibility. Officials from Florida told us that their AVS is connected to the vast majority of banks operating in their state. Although all states were required to have an electronic AVS in place by the end of fiscal year 2013,[57] only 2 of the 12 states for which we conducted interviews reported having implemented an AVS. In our prior work, we found that states identified challenges to implementing an AVS, including a lack of resources—money, staff, or time—to implement the system, and challenges getting financial institutions to participate.[58]

Eligibility workers from one county reported using certain commercial investigative software that pulls together publically available information nationwide to help verify or identify applicants' assets or transfers. This software can help eligibility workers find information on unreported assets and transfers, such as information about property deeds or ownership of a business. The workers reported that this software is used in cases where the eligibility worker suspects the applicant owns, for example, an out-of-state unreported asset. In this county, only the two eligibility worker supervisors and investigative staff have access to this software.

AGENCY COMMENTS

We provided a draft of this report to HHS for review. HHS had no general comments but provided technical comments that we incorporated as appropriate.

Carolyn L. Yocom
Director, Health Care

APPENDIX I: SUMMARY OF APPLICATION FILES REVIEWED IN SELECTED COUNTIES IN THREE STATES

Of the 350 Medicaid applicants whose files we reviewed in selected counties in three states (Florida, New York, and South Carolina), most were over 75 years old, single, and female. (See table 6.) The median age of applicants was 84 years old. A majority of applicants—80 percent—had been living in a long-term care facility, such as a nursing home, at the time they applied for Medicaid coverage of nursing home care. The median length of time these applicants had been living in facilities was 2.3 months; the length of time ranged from less than 1 month to 6 years. Some applicants—15 percent—were already covered under Medicaid for basic medical services at the time that they applied for coverage of nursing home care. Additionally, 24 percent of the applicants had evidence in their application file that they received assistance from an attorney or financial planner in applying for Medicaid coverage for nursing home care. Over 80 percent of the applicants whose files we reviewed (294 of 350) were approved for Medicaid coverage for nursing home care, while 15 percent of applicants (52 of 350) were initially denied Medicaid coverage. (See fig. 5.) Most of these applicants (39 of 52) were denied because they failed to provide required documentation, a few were denied because they were not functionally eligible (4 of 52), and some applicants (11 of 52) were denied for financial reasons, including having income or resources that exceeded financial eligibility standards.[1] For applicants denied for having excess income, the median amount of excess income was $77 per month; for those denied for excess resources, the median amount of excess resources was $20,407.[2] Most applicants (9 of 11) who were initially denied for financial reasons reapplied and were later approved for

Table 6. Characteristics of Applicants Reviewed in Selected Counties in Three States (n=350)

Characteristic	Number of applicants	Percent of applicants
Age		
65 to 69	29	8
70 to 74	38	11
75 to 79	48	14
80 to 84	68	19
85 to 89	87	25
90 and older Gender[a]	80	23
Female	234	67
Male	114	33
Marital status		
Married	88	25
Single	262	75
Living in long-term care facility at time of application	278	80

Source: GAO analysis of Medicaid application data.

Note: Data for four counties were from applications submitted during state fiscal year 2012, while data for two counties were from applications submitted between July 1, 2012, and December 31, 2012.

[a]We did not have information on the gender of two applicants.

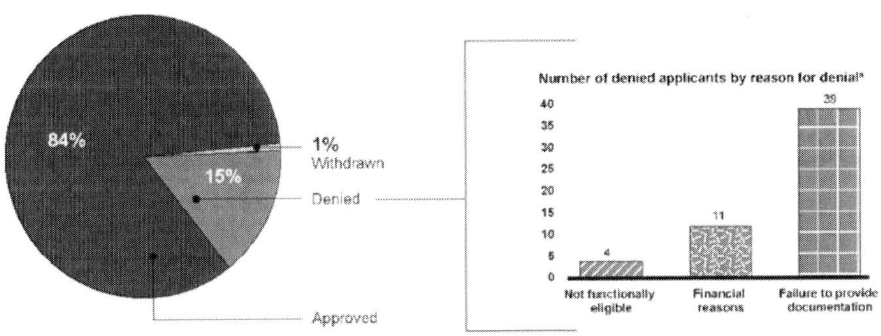

Source: GAO analysis of Medicaid application data.

Notes: Data for four counties were from applications submitted during state fiscal year 2012, while data for two counties were from applications submitted between July 1, 2012, and December 31, 2012.

[a]A total of 52 of the 350 applicants whose files we reviewed were denied. However, three applicants were denied for more than one reason and are included in the count for both categories for which they were denied.

Figure 5. Application Status of Medicaid Applicants Reviewed in Selected Counties in Three States (n=350).

Medicaid coverage for nursing home care. Of the 9 applicants who were later approved for Medicaid, 3 applicants spent down assets on long-term care or medical expenses, 2 applicants spent down assets on other goods or services, 2 applicants placed excess income into a qualified income trust, and 2 applicants were later approved for other or unknown reasons.

APPENDIX II: SCOPE AND METHODOLOGY

To examine the financial characteristics of applicants approved for Medicaid nursing home coverage, we reviewed a random sample of Medicaid nursing home application files in selected counties in three states. To select states, we used information from a 2011 GAO web-based survey of Medicaid officials from each of the 50 states and the District of Columbia.[1] We scored states based on their survey responses to questions on the extent to which they:

1) verify applicants' assets with financial institutions;
2) conduct property record searches; and
3) obtain information covering the 60-month look-back period.

Weighing each question equally, we ranked states on the basis of their total score and placed them into three groups (low, medium, and high) using naturally occurring breaks in the data. (See table 7.) In selecting states, we considered the geographic dispersion of states, as well as the following:

- among states in the "low" group, we focused on states that reported generally obtaining only 1 month of documentation; and
- among states in the "high" group, we focused on states that reported conducting all three activities to some extent—verifying assets with financial institutions, conducting property searches, and obtaining 60 months of documentation.

From the ranked group of low and high states, we selected an initial set of states plus additional alternative states, and conducted interviews with state officials to determine whether they could provide us with needed data in order to select a sample of counties and application files to review.[2] If a state informed us they were unable to provide such data, we replaced the state with the next alternative state from the respective group. We interviewed officials from a total of 11 states. Officials from 6 states (2 high and 4 low) told us they were unable to produce needed data due to data system limitations. Officials from 1 state (a high state) told us they were technically able to produce needed data but would not be able to do so within a reasonable timeframe due to competing demands for their information technology resources. This left us with 4 states—2 high states and 2 low states—that were able to produce the data we needed. Based on these interviews, we selected one state from the low group (Florida) and two states from the high group (New York and South Carolina). In 2012, Medicaid spending for institutional longterm care was $3.3 billion in Florida, $11.5 billion in New York, and $801 million in South Carolina.

Table 7. Groups Used for State Sample Selection

Group	Total Number of States	States
Low	14	Arizona, Arkansas, California, District of Columbia, Florida, Idaho, Massachusetts, Minnesota, Nebraska, New Mexico, North Dakota, Tennessee, Virginia, West Virginia
Medium	22	Alaska, Colorado, Delaware, Georgia, Illinois, Indiana, Iowa, Kansas, Kentucky, Louisiana, Michigan, Mississippi, Ohio, Oklahoma, Oregon, Pennsylvania, South Dakota,Texas, Utah, Washington, Wisconsin, Wyoming
High	15	Alabama, Connecticut, Hawaii, Maine, Maryland, Missouri, Montana, Nevada, New Hampshire, New Jersey, New York, North Carolina, Rhode Island, South Carolina, Vermont

Source: GAO survey of Medicaid officials in 50 states and the District of Columbia, 2011.

To choose counties in our selected states, we considered three factors.

1) Size of the population aged 65 and older.[3]
2) Median income of households with householders aged 65 and older.[4]
3) Number of Medicaid nursing home applications received.[5]

For the three factors, we ranked the counties within each selected state from high to low. We chose two counties that appeared in the top 20 ranking for all three factors in Florida,[6] or the top 10 ranking for all three factors in New York and South Carolina. (See table 8.)

Table 8. Selected States and Counties

Selected states	Selected counties
Florida	Palm Beach and Sarasota
South Carolina	Charleston and Richland
New York	Nassau and Westchester

Source: GAO.

Each selected state sent us a list of individuals aged 65 or over who submitted an application for Medicaid coverage for nursing home care during our requested time period in our selected counties—for Florida and South Carolina, we received a list of applicants who applied for services from July 1, 2011, through June 30, 2012, and for New York, we received a list of applicants who applied from July 1, 2012, through December 31, 2012. From the lists provided by the states, we randomly selected application files. In order to compensate for application files that would need to be skipped because we determined that they did not meet our criteria or lacked adequate information, we requested additional files in each county. When we determined that an application file was unusable, we included the next application file on our randomly generated list.

We based the number of application files selected for review in each county on the total number of Medicaid nursing home applications that the county received from applicants aged 65 and older during our requested time period. We reviewed a total of 350 nursing home application files, of which 294 were approved for Medicaid coverage of nursing home care, including those that were approved and incurred a penalty period. (See table 9.)

Table 9. Number of Files Reviewed, by Selected State and County

Selected state	Selected county	Total number of files reviewed	Number of approved files reviewed
Florida	Palm Beach	67	53
	Sarasota	59	53
	Total	126	106
New York	Nassau	57	50
	Westchester	57	40
	Total	114	90
South Carolina	Charleston	52	47
	Richland	58	51
	Total	110	98
Total		350	294

Source: GAO.

We established a file review protocol whereby we reviewed and recorded the earliest Medicaid application for nursing home care in each file during the requested time period. If this application was denied, then we recorded data from that application, as well as certain data from the last application subsequently submitted by the time in which we reviewed files, if there was one. From each application, we collected and analyzed data on the amount and type of applicants' income and resources, including both countable and noncountable resources; certain applicant demographic information, such as marital status; and whether applicants were found to have transferred assets for less than fair market value (FMV) during the look-back period, how the assets were transferred, and the value of the assets transferred.

Since the selected counties used the information in these application files to determine eligibility for Medicaid coverage for nursing home care, we did not independently verify the accuracy of the information contained in the files. However, to ensure that the information we entered into our data collection instrument was consistent with the information found in the application files, we conducted independent file verifications, which resulted in verification of at least 20 percent of the files reviewed. For some applicants, while the application file noted the applicant had income from a certain source or owned a certain type of resource, the amount of income or value of the resource was missing. This missing information may have affected the distributions of applicants by their amount of income or resources, as well as the medians, averages, and ranges of income and resources we report. Where applicable, we provide information on the extent of missing information in our analysis. Additionally, we conducted electronic tests of the data collected to determine whether there were obvious errors. In some cases, we combined variables to create new ones. For example, we collected and identified several types of applicant resources, but ultimately combined them into two categories—total resources and noncountable resources. Based on these procedures, we determined that the data were sufficiently reliable for the purposes of this report. The data from the 294 approved application files cannot be generalized to other approved applicants.

To identify the methods used to reduce countable assets to qualify for Medicaid coverage for nursing home care, we reviewed applicable federal laws and guidance, and spoke with officials from the Centers for Medicare & Medicaid Services (CMS), the agency within the Department of Health and Human Services (HHS) that oversees the Medicaid program. We also used information from the following sources:

- Interviews with attorneys: We interviewed 9 of 16 attorneys recommended to us by the Director of the American Bar Association's Commission on Law and Aging. To select among the recommended attorneys, we considered the state in which the attorney practiced and our previously established grouping of the extent to which states take steps to verify applicants' assets. We selected attorneys from each group and from as many different states as possible, including states where we conducted file reviews.
- Undercover calls with law office representatives: We conducted undercover calls with representatives from a selection of law offices whose websites indicated that they offered Medicaid planning services for elderly individuals.[7] We contacted 36 law offices for the undercover calls and determined 17 of the calls to be successful—that is, an attorney or another representative was willing to provide information over the phone and free of charge.[8] During the calls, our investigator used one of three scenarios in which he posed as an adult child seeking advice on ways in which he could obtain Medicaid coverage for nursing home care for his parent, while preserving the parent's assets for a spouse or heirs. The different scenarios created were intended to test for potential differences in planning methods based on marital status and the timing of the need for nursing home care. Two scenarios involved an elderly parent with an immediate need for care (one for a married individual and one for a widow) and the third scenario involved an elderly parent for whom the need for long-term care services was not immediate, but would likely occur sometime in the future (possibly beyond the 60-month look-back period).
- Interviews with state Medicaid officials: We interviewed state Medicaid officials from the 3 states in which we reviewed files, as well as 9 additional states (for a total of 12 states) about the methods used by applicants in their state to reduce countable assets, and any steps that the state has taken to try to alleviate or eliminate the use of such methods. We selected the states based on information collected from our calls with attorneys, undercover calls with representatives from law offices, information from background literature, and data on the percentage of the population aged 65 and older and the percentage of elderly (age 65 and older) with income at or above 150 percent of the poverty level. We also considered geographic variation. The 12 states from which we interviewed Medicaid officials were: Colorado,

Connecticut, Florida, Massachusetts, Michigan, New Jersey, New York, Ohio, Rhode Island, South Carolina, Vermont, and Washington.

- Interviews with county eligibility workers: We conducted in-person, semi-structured group interviews with eligibility workers from two counties from the three states in which we conducted file reviews, as well as from three additional states.[9] To select the three additional states, we used information from interviews with attorneys, undercover calls with representatives from law offices, and literature. We also took into consideration geographic distribution of states. To choose counties in the additional states, we ranked the counties in each state based on the size of the population aged 65 and older,[10] and median income of households with householders aged 65 and older.[11]

In addition, where feasible, we used information collected from our review of Medicaid nursing home application files to supplement the information obtained from our interviews and undercover calls.

To identify the information eligibility workers considered the most useful for identifying and verifying applicants' financial eligibility, we used information from the interviews conducted with county eligibility workers in two counties in six states.

We conducted this performance audit from September 2012 to May 2014 in accordance with generally accepted government auditing standards. Those standards require that we plan and perform the audit to obtain sufficient, appropriate evidence to provide a reasonable basis for our findings and conclusions based on our audit objectives. We believe that the evidence obtained provides a reasonable basis for our findings and conclusions based on our audit objectives. We conducted our related investigative work in accordance with investigation standards prescribed by the Council of the Inspectors General on Integrity and Efficiency.

End Notes

[1] MetLife Mature Market Institute, *Market Survey of Long-Term Care Costs* (New York, N.Y.: November 2012). In addition to nursing home services, other health care services for long-term care include home health, personal care services, assisted living, and noninstitutional group living arrangements.

[2] Assets include income, which is anything received during a calendar month that is used or could be used to meet food or shelter needs; and resources, which are anything owned, such as bank accounts or property, that can be converted to cash. This terminology is based on

definitions provided in *The State Medicaid Manual* issued by the Centers for Medicare & Medicaid Services, which specifies that assets include both income and resources.

[3] This report focuses on financial eligibility. Individuals applying for Medicaid coverage for long-term care must also meet functional eligibility criteria established by each state. Functional eligibility criteria generally involve a degree of impairment measured by limitations in an individual's ability to carry out certain activities of daily living, such as eating and dressing; and instrumental activities of daily living, such as preparing meals and grocery shopping.

[4] GAO, *Medicaid Long-Term Care: Information Obtained by States About Applicants' Assets Varies and May Be Insufficient*, GAO-12-749 (Washington, D.C.: July 26, 2012).

[5] GAO, *Medicaid Long-Term Care: Few Transferred Assets Before Applying for Nursing Home Coverage; Impact of Deficit Reduction Act on Eligibility is Uncertain*, GAO-07-280 (Washington, D.C.: Mar. 26, 2007).

[6] GAO, *Medicaid: Transfers of Assets by Elderly Individuals to Obtain Long-Term Care Coverage,* GAO-05-968 (Washington, D.C.: Sept. 2, 2005).

[7] See Pub. L. No. 109-171, §§ 6011-6016, 120 Stat. 4, 61-67 (2006).

[8] The three actions were the extent to which states reported they (1) verified applicants' assets with financial institutions; (2) conducted property record searches; and (3) obtained information covering the 60-month look-back period. See GAO-12-749 for the results of this survey.

[9] The applications reviewed were of individuals aged 65 or older at the time they applied for Medicaid nursing home coverage. In Florida and South Carolina, we reviewed applications submitted in the state fiscal year ending in 2012 (July 1, 2011, through June 30, 2012). In New York, we reviewed applications submitted between July 1, 2012, and December 31, 2012, due to limitations in the state's data systems prior to that date.

[10] Not all SSI recipients automatically qualify for Medicaid. Under Section 1902(f) of the Social Security Act, a state may use more restrictive Medicaid eligibility standards than SSI's standards, provided the standards are no more restrictive than those the state had in place as of January 1, 1972. As of March 2013, 11 states had opted to use these standards. These states are often referred to as 209(b) states because the origin of this provision was § 209(b) of the Social Security Amendments of 1972, Pub. L. No. 92-603, 86 Stat. 1329, 1381.

[11] Medicaid and CHIP Payment and Access Commission, *Report to the Congress on Medicaid and CHIP, March 2013* (Washington, D.C.: Mar. 15, 2013).

[12] Medicaid and CHIP Payment and Access Commission, *Report to Congress, March 2013.*

[13] Money from this irrevocable trust is used to pay for specific costs, such as the applicant's care. Following the individual's death, the state receives all remaining amounts in this trust up to the amount spent by the state for the individual's care.

[14] See 42 U.S.C. § 1396p(d)(4)(B).

[15] An individual with substantial home equity is not excluded from eligibility for Medicaid payment for long-term care if a spouse, child under age 21, or child who is considered blind or disabled lives in the home. 42 U.S.C. § 1396p(f)(2).

[16] 42 U.S.C. § 1396r-5.

[17] If one-half of a couple's combined countable resources is less than a state-specified minimum resource level, then the community spouse may retain resources up to the minimum level. States' minimum resource levels cannot be less than the federal minimum resource standard, which was $23,448 for 2014.

[18] We use community spouse resource allowance to refer to the amount of a couple's combined jointly and separately-owned resources allocated to the community spouse and considered

unavailable to the institutionalized spouse when determining his or her eligibility for Medicaid.

[19] The Social Security Act terms this the minimum monthly maintenance needs allowance. Throughout this report, we refer to this as the minimum needs allowance.

[20] If the institutionalized spouse's income is not sufficient to make up the difference, then the community spouse would be allowed to keep resources above the community spouse resource allowance, so that the additional resources could be used to generate more income.

[21] Per federal standards, as of January 1, 2014, the minimum needs allowance for Alaska must be at least $2,422.50 and for Hawaii must be at least $2,231.25.

[22] Federal law requires states to apply the transfer of asset provisions to institutionalized individuals, who are defined in the Social Security Act as individuals who are inpatients in a nursing facility or in a medical institution that is being paid based on a level of care received in a nursing home, or certain recipients of home and community-based services. 42 U.S.C. § 1396p(h)(3). States have the option to apply such provisions to noninstitutionalized individuals.

[23] The length of the penalty period, in months, is calculated by dividing the total cumulative amount of assets transferred for less than FMV by the average monthly private pay rate for nursing home care in the state (or the community in which the applicant is institutionalized, at the option of the state).

[24] Additional exemptions from the penalty period include transfers of assets to an individual for the spouse's sole benefit or to a trust for a disabled child's sole benefit. Transfers of a home are also exempt if made to an individual's spouse, or minor or disabled child; an adult child residing in the home who has been caring for the individual for a specified time period; or a sibling who has an equity interest in the home and has resided in the individual's home for at least 1 year immediately prior to the date the individual became institutionalized. 42 U.S.C. § 1396p(c)(2)(A)-(c)(2)(B).

[25] Transfers also do not result in a penalty when the individual can show that he or she intended to dispose of the assets at FMV or for other valuable consideration, or that all assets transferred for less than FMV have been returned to the individual. 42 U.S.C. § 1396p(c)(2)(C).

[26] For additional information on the extent to which states require individuals applying for Medicaid coverage for long-term care to document assets and obtain information about these applicants' assets from third parties, see GAO-12-749.

[27] For two approved applicants who owned at least one resource, there was no information available on the value of any of their resources. As such, the percentages presented do not add up to 100 percent.

[28] Total resources of approved applicants averaged $60,375 and ranged from $0 to $1,551,344.

[29] The median net worth of elderly households in the United States was $170,516 in 2011. Net worth is defined as the total value of all of the resources that an individual or household owns, including the value of real estate, stocks, bonds, retirement accounts, and other resources, minus debts or liabilities. Elderly households are those with a householder aged 65 or older; the householder is the person in whose name the home is owned or rented. See U.S. Census Bureau, *Survey of Income and Program Participation, 2008 Panel, Wave 10*, accessed March 28, 2014, http://www.census.gov/people/wealth/files/Wealth_Tables_2011.xlsx.

[30] Total resources for approved applicants who were married averaged $169,968 and ranged from $0 to $1,551,344; for single applicants, total resources averaged $25,822 and ranged from $0 to $460,147.

[31] Twenty-three approved applicants whose files we reviewed owned at least one noncountable resource but there was no information available on the value of any of the noncountable resources that they owned.

[32] Noncountable resources for approved applicants averaged $80,427 and ranged from $0 to $1,541,565.

[33] Noncountable resources for approved applicants who were married averaged $180,594 and ranged from $12 to $1,541,565; for single applicants, noncountable resources averaged $36,972 and ranged from $0 to $446,166.

[34] The amount of allowable home equity interest is established by each state within federal guidelines and could range from $543,000 to $814,000 in 2014. However, an individual with home equity greater than the state's allowable amount is not excluded from eligibility if a spouse, child under age 21, or child who is blind or disabled lives in the home.

[35] In Florida and South Carolina, applicants can place income above the special income level for nursing home residents in a qualified income trust, which is used to pay for the applicants' care. New York has a "medically needy" option, whereby applicants can qualify for coverage if their income, after subtracting any medical expenses, is less than or equal to the state's income standard.

[36] Annual gross income for all approved applicants averaged $20,607 and ranged from $360 to $161,064.

[37] The median annual income of the elderly in the United States was $20,308 ($2,828 per month) in 2012. See U.S. Census Bureau, *Current Population Survey, 2013 Annual Social and Economic Supplements*, accessed April 1, 2014, http://www.census.gov/hhes/www/cpstables/032013/perinc/pinc02_000.htm.

[38] The average amount of approved applicants' income that was provided to the community spouse was $1,186 per month, and the amount ranged from $178 to $3,535 per month. Applicant files for five married applicants did not indicate whether income from the institutionalized spouse was provided to the community spouse.

[39] Applicants in South Carolina and New York were subject to a 60-month look-back period. Florida, however, did not implement the DRA provision to extend the look-back period from 36 months to 60 months until 2010, after which it was phased in over time. As a result, applicants whose files we reviewed in Florida were subject to a 36-month look-back period.

[40] Irrevocable means that the annuity cannot be changed or terminated, and nonassignable means that the annuity cannot be transferred to another individual. As previously noted, the DRA specified that annuities purchased by or on behalf of the individual applying for Medicaid must meet criteria such as being actuarially sound—that is, they must pay out during the applicant's life expectancy; providing payments in equal amounts during the term of the annuity; and naming the state as the primary remainder beneficiary unless there is a community spouse or minor or disabled child. Otherwise, the annuity would be considered a transfer for less than FMV.

[41] A promissory note is a written, unconditional agreement, usually given in return for goods, money loaned, or services rendered, whereby one party promises to pay a certain sum of money at a specified time (or on demand) to another party.

[42] The purchase of a promissory note is to be considered a transfer for less than FMV unless the repayment terms are actuarially sound, it provides for payments to be made in equal amounts during the term of the loan with no deferral or balloon payments, and it prohibits the cancellation of the balance upon the death of the lender. 42 U.S.C. § 1396p(c)(1)(I).

[43] For example, if the applicant transferred $35,000 worth of assets for less than FMV and the average monthly private pay rate for nursing home care in the state was $7,000, the penalty period would be 5 months.

[44] As we previously reported, prior to the DRA, individuals used a mechanism commonly referred to as the "half-a-loaf" strategy, which involved transferring a portion (e.g., half) of one's assets and waiting out a penalty period before applying for Medicaid coverage of nursing home care. However, the DRA changes to the start date of the penalty period eliminated the availability of the "half-a-loaf" strategy. According to state Medicaid officials and attorneys we spoke with, the "reverse half-a-loaf" mechanism has since emerged.

[45] If all of the transferred assets are returned, then the penalty period is eliminated. However, the returned assets will likely be considered countable assets for purposes of determining the individual's Medicaid eligibility.

[46] Generally, when an applicant assigns his or her support rights to a state, the state supports and pays for the medical care of the applicant. In exchange, the applicant agrees to cooperate in providing information and assisting the state in pursuing support from the community spouse.

[47] Under federal law, an institutionalized spouse cannot be considered financially ineligible due to excess resources if one of the following three conditions are met: (1) the institutionalized spouse has assigned to the state their rights to support from the community spouse; (2) the institutionalized spouse lacks the ability to execute an assignment of support rights due to physical or mental impairment, but the state has the right to sue the community spouse for support without such assignment; or (3) the state has determined that denial of eligibility would result in an undue hardship to the institutionalized spouse. 42 U.S.C. § 1396r-5(c)(3).

[48] The average amount of nonhousing resources the community spouse retained was $436,949, and ranged from $13,306 to $1,585,467. According the federal standards, the maximum amount of countable resources that a community spouse can retain is $117,240 in 2014. That amount was $113,640 in 2012.

[49] The amount of monthly income support provided to the community spouse averaged $1,416 and ranged from $441 to $2,088.

[50] Per federal law, a month after eligibility is determined, and during the continuous period in which the institutionalized spouse remains in an institution, the community spouse's resources are deemed unavailable and thus not countable. 42 U.S.C § 1396r-5(c)(4).

[51] 42 U.S.C. § 1396r-5(d)(4).

[52] GAO-12-749.

[53] GAO-12-749.

[54] GAO-12-749.

[55] In 2008, Congress passed legislation that required states to implement electronic AVS to verify the assets of aged, blind, or disabled applicants for Medicaid, including those seeking Medicaid coverage for long-term care, with financial institutions. Supplemental Appropriations Act, 2008, Pub. L. No. 110-252, § 7001(d)(1), 122 Stat. 2323, 2391 (codified at 42 U.S.C. § 1396w).

[56] Florida began a pilot of its AVS in selected counties in October 2012, and implemented the program statewide in February 2013.

[57] The Supplemental Appropriations Act, 2008, required California, New Jersey, and New York to implement an AVS for aged, blind, and disabled applicants by the end of fiscal year 2009, and directed the Secretary of HHS to require the remaining states to implement their systems in a manner that results in a specified percentage of aged, blind, and disabled

Medicaid applicants being subject to this type of asset verification each year of the 5-year period from fiscal year 2009 through fiscal year 2013.

[58] GAO-12-749.

End Notes for Appendix I

[1] Three applicants were denied for more than one reason.

[2] The amount of excess income averaged $166 per month and ranged from $9 to $412 per month. The amount of excess resources averaged $59,063 and ranged from $7,964 to $182,649.

End Notes for Appendix II

[1] GAO, *Medicaid Long-Term Care: Information Obtained by States about Applicants' Assets Varies and May be Insufficient,* GAO-12-749 (Washington, D.C.: July 26, 2012). The survey requested information about the types of documentation, if any, that states require applicants for Medicaid coverage for long-term care to submit for 13 types of assets: (1) earned income, (2) unearned income, (3) financial and investment resources, (4) life insurance, (5) primary residence, (6) real property other than primary residence, (7) vehicles, (8) annuities, (9) burial contracts and prepaid funeral arrangements, (10) continuing care retirement community entrance fees, (11) life estates, (12) promissory notes or loans, and (13) trusts. In addition, the survey asked about the number of months of documentation states required for earned income, unearned income, and financial and investment resources. The survey also asked about states' practices to obtain information from third parties to verify applicants' assets, such as whether, and to what extent, states conduct data matches with 10 sources, including the Social Security Administration and the Internal Revenue Service, which primarily allow states to verify applicants' income. Finally, the survey asked about any additional documentation states require or additional steps states take to determine whether applicants transferred assets for less than fair market value during the 60-month look-back period.

[2] In making this selection, we excluded some states, such as states that had smaller populations, states that had lower median incomes among the population aged 65 and older; and states that, to our knowledge, had not implemented the Deficit Reduction Act of 2005 by our time period of interest, which was generally state fiscal year 2012.

[3] We used information from the *Profile of General Population and Housing Characteristics: 2010*, U.S. Census Bureau.

[4] We used information from the *Median Household Income in the Past 12 Months (in 2010 Inflation-Adjusted Dollars) by Age of Householder*, U.S. Census Bureau, 2006-2010 American Community Survey.

[5] We used information provided by state officials in each of the three states. For Florida and South Carolina, we used data on the number of applications received for Medicaid coverage for nursing home services from individuals aged 65 and older from July 1, 2011, through June 30, 2012. Due to limitations in New York's data systems, we used data on the number of applications received for Medicaid coverage for nursing home services from individuals aged 65 and older from July 1, 2012, through December 31, 2012.

[6] No counties in Florida were in the top 10 for all three factors.

[7] To identify these professionals, we conducted an Internet search using search terms related to Medicaid planning and long-term care to identify attorneys or financial planners that offered Medicaid planning services for elderly individuals. We took the first 100 results from the search, all of which were law offices, and selected offices to contact based on the services they advertised providing, and taking into consideration geographic variation. In case some law offices were not responsive to our inquiry, we had a methodology for selecting alternatives to ensure continued geographic variation.

[8] We considered our contacts with the other 19 law offices as unsuccessful for the following reasons: the office informed us that they required a fee for consultation, an in-person consultation, or both (10 offices); the office informed us that they were unable to provide assistance, but could provide a referral to someone else (2 offices); or we were unable to make contact with the office after repeated contact attempts (7 offices).

[9] We requested that the eligibility workers interviewed had reviewed Medicaid long-term care applications for at least 12 months, were considered specialists in Medicaid longterm care applications or primarily process these types of applications, and were not supervisors.

[10] We used information from the *Profile of General Population and Housing Characteristics: 2010*, U.S. Census Bureau.

[11] We used information from the *Median Household Income in the Past 12 Months (in 2010 Inflation-Adjusted Dollars) by Age of Householder*, U.S. Census Bureau, 2006-2010 American Community Survey.

In: Medicaid and Long-Term Care Assistance ISBN: 978-1-63463-328-4
Editor: Corynn D. Ford

Chapter 3

MEDICAID: AN OVERVIEW*

Alison Mitchell, Evelyne P. Baumrucker and Elicia J. Hgberz

SUMMARY

Medicaid is a means-tested entitlement program that in FY2012 financed the delivery of primary and acute medical services as well as long-term services and supports to an estimated 57 million people, and cost states and the federal government $431 billion. In comparison, the Medicare program provided health care benefits to nearly 50 million seniors and certain individuals with disabilities in FY2012 at a cost of roughly $557 billion. Because Medicaid represents a large component of federal mandatory spending, Congress is likely to continue its oversight of Medicaid's eligibility, benefits, and costs.

Participation in Medicaid is voluntary for states, though all states, the District of Columbia, and U.S. territories choose to participate. In order to participate in Medicaid, the federal government requires states to cover certain mandatory populations and benefits, but the federal government also allows states to cover other optional populations and services. Due to this flexibility, there is substantial variation among the states in terms of factors such as Medicaid eligibility, covered benefits, and provider payment rates. In addition, there are several waiver and demonstration

---

* This is an edited, reformatted and augmented version of a Congressional Research Service publication, No. R43357, dated January 10, 2014.

authorities that allow states to operate their Medicaid program outside of federal rules.

Historically, Medicaid eligibility has generally been limited to low-income children, pregnant women, parents of dependent children, the elderly, and individuals with disabilities; however, the Patient Protection and Affordable Care Act (ACA; P.L. 111-148, as amended) included the ACA Medicaid expansion, which expands Medicaid eligibility to individuals under the age of 65 with income up to 133% of the federal poverty level (FPL) (effectively 138% FPL) at state option.

The ACA makes a number of other changes, which together represent the most significant reform to the Medicaid program since its establishment in 1965. In addition to the ACA Medicaid expansion, the ACA also expands Medicaid eligibility for children ages 6 to 18 and former foster care children; transitions to the modified adjusted gross income (MAGI) counting methodology for most nonelderly Medicaid enrollees; requires alternative benefit plan (ABP) coverage for certain Medicaid enrollees; provides enhanced federal matching funds for the ACA Medicaid expansion; increases uniformity among Medicare, Medicaid, and the State Children's Health Insurance Program (CHIP) program integrity activities; and provides the Centers for Medicare & Medicaid Services (CMS) with the ability to test methods to improve coordination of care for dual-eligible beneficiaries, among a number of other changes.

This report describes the basic elements of Medicaid, focusing on who is eligible, what services are covered, how enrollees share in the cost of care, how the program is financed, and how providers are paid. The report also explains waivers, program integrity activities, and the dual-eligible population. In addition, the report describes the following selected issues: the ACA Medicaid expansion, the impact of the ACA health insurance annual fee on Medicaid, and the ACA maintenance of effort (MOE) with respect to Medicaid eligibility.

INTRODUCTION

Medicaid is a joint federal-state program that finances the delivery of primary and acute medical services, as well as LTSS, for a diverse low-income population, including children, pregnant women, adults, individuals with chronic disabling conditions, and people age 65 and older. In FY2012, Medicaid is estimated to have provided health care services to 56.7 million individuals[1] at a total cost of $431 billion, with the federal government paying $249 billion (about 58%) of that total.[2]

Medicaid is an important health care safety net[3] for low-income populations with approximately 18% of the U.S. population enrolled in Medicaid in CY2011.[4] For some types of services, Medicaid is a significant payer. For instance, in CY2011, Medicaid accounted for 42% of national spending on long-term services and supports (LTSS) and 25% of all mental health and substance abuse treatment spending.[5] Also, along with the State Children's Health Insurance Program (CHIP), Medicaid paid for almost half of all births in the United States (about 1.8 million hospital births) in 2010.[6]

Medicaid is one of the largest payers in the U.S. health care system, representing 15.1% of national health care spending in calendar year (CY) 2011; in that year, private health insurance and Medicare accounted for 33.2% and 20.5%, respectively.[7]

Medicaid was enacted in 1965 as part of the same law that created the Medicare program (the Social Security Amendments of 1965; P.L. 89-97). State participation in Medicaid is voluntary, though all states, the District of Columbia, and the territories[8] choose to participate. States are responsible for administering their Medicaid programs. Medicaid is jointly financed by the federal government and the states. Federal Medicaid spending is an entitlement,[9] with total expenditures dependent on state policy decisions and use of services by enrollees.

States must follow broad federal rules in order to receive federal matching funds, but have flexibility to design their own version of Medicaid within the federal statute's basic framework. This flexibility results in variability across state Medicaid programs. Each state has a Medicaid state plan that describes how the state will administer its Medicaid program. States submit these Medicaid state plans to the federal Centers for Medicare and Medicaid Services (CMS) for approval.[10]

Medicaid was designed to provide coverage to groups with a wide range of health care needs who were historically excluded from the private health insurance market (e.g., individuals with chronic disabling conditions who require LTSS or indigent populations in geographic locations where access to providers is limited). Because of the diversity of the populations that Medicaid serves, Medicaid offers some benefits that are not typically covered by major insurance plans offered in the private market (e.g., nursing facility care or early and periodic screening, diagnosis, and treatment [EPSDT] services).[11] Medicaid also pays for Medicare premiums and/or cost sharing for low-income seniors and individuals with disabilities, who are eligible for both programs, referred to as dual-eligible beneficiaries. For other Medicaid enrollees, out-of-pocket costs are generally nominal, which may not be the case with most employer-sponsored or exchange health insurance coverage.[12] The Medicaid program pays for special classes of providers, such as federally qualified health centers (FQHCs), rural health clinics (RHCs), and Indian Health Service (IHS) facilities, that provide health care services to populations in areas where access to traditional physician care has been limited.

Since its inception, the Medicaid program has expanded in a number of different directions. Federal laws have changed virtually every aspect of the program, affecting eligibility, benefits, beneficiary cost-sharing, and fraud and abuse protections, among others. The Patient Protection and Affordable Care Act (ACA; P.L. 111-148 as amended) is the most recent federal law to make fundamental revisions to the Medicaid program, including a substantial expansion of Medicaid eligibility, beginning in 2014. The ACA will likely broaden Medicaid's role in providing health care coverage to the U.S. population, and increase the likelihood that, going forward, Congress's attention to health policy issues will involve Medicaid.

The ACA was designed to reduce the number of U.S. citizens without health insurance by preserving the existing system of employer-based health insurance, making changes to the individual insurance market, and expanding coverage to the uninsured through Medicaid and health insurance exchanges (also referred to as marketplaces).[13] Under the ACA, Medicaid and the exchanges are envisioned to work in tandem to provide a continuous source of subsidized coverage for lower-income individuals and families.[14] Medicaid agencies are required to coordinate with the exchanges to educate people about new health insurance options and assist them in navigating the enrollment process.

This report describes the basic elements of Medicaid, focusing on who is eligible, what services are covered, how enrollees share in the cost of care, how the program is financed, and how providers are paid. The report also explains waivers, program integrity activities, and the dual-eligible population. In addition, the report describes the following selected issues: the ACA Medicaid expansion, the impact of the ACA health insurance annual fee on Medicaid, and the ACA maintenance of effort (MOE) with respect to Medicaid eligibility.

ELIGIBILITY

Eligibility for Medicaid is determined by both federal and state law, whereby states set individual eligibility criteria within federal minimum standards. Individuals must meet both *categorical* (e.g., elderly, individuals with disabilities, children, pregnant women, parents, certain nonelderly childless adults) and *financial* (i.e., income and sometimes assets limits) criteria.[15] In addition, individuals need to meet federal and state requirements regarding residency, immigration status, and documentation of U.S. citizenship. Some eligibility groups are mandatory, meaning that all states with a Medicaid program must cover them; others are optional. States are permitted to apply to CMS for a waiver of federal law to expand health coverage beyond the mandatory and optional groups listed in federal statute (see the "Medicaid Program Waivers" section for more information about waivers).

If a state participates in Medicaid, the following are examples of groups that *must* be provided Medicaid coverage:

- poor families that meet the financial requirements (based on family size) of the former Aid to Families with Dependent Children (AFDC) cash assistance program;
- pregnant women and children through age 18 with family income at or below 133% of the federal poverty level (FPL);[16]
- low-income individuals who are age 65 and older, or blind, or who are under age 65 and disabled who qualify for cash assistance under the Supplemental Security Income (SSI) program;
- recipients of adoption assistance and foster care (who are under age 18) under Title IV–E of the Social Security Act;
- certain individuals who age out of foster care, up to age 26, and do not qualify under other mandatory groups noted above; and
- certain groups of legal permanent resident immigrants (e.g., refugees for the first seven years after entry into the United States; asylees for the first seven years after asylum is granted; lawful permanent aliens with 40 quarters of creditable coverage under Social Security; immigrants who are honorably discharged U.S. military veterans) who meet all other financial and categorical Medicaid eligibility requirements.

Examples of groups that states *may* provide Medicaid to include

- pregnant women and infants with family income between 133% and 185% of the FPL;

- certain individuals who qualify for nursing facility or other institutional care and have incomes up to 300% of SSI benefit level, referred to as "the 300 percent rule";
- "medically needy" individuals who are members of one of the broad categories of Medicaid covered groups (i.e., are aged, have a disability, or are in families with children), but do not meet the applicable income requirements and, in some instances, assets requirements for those eligibility pathways;[17] and
- working people with disabilities.

Beginning in 2014, states have the option to expand Medicaid eligibility beyond the historical categorical eligibility groups to all citizens under age 65, who otherwise are not eligible for Medicaid with income at or below 133% of FPL (i.e., the ACA Medicaid expansion). The income limit is effectively 138% of FPL (after adjusting for a 5% income disregard applicable if individuals are at the highest income limits for coverage).[18] (For more information about the ACA Medicaid expansion, see "ACA Medicaid Expansion.")

Modified Adjusted Gross Income (MAGI)

As of January 1, 2014, the modified adjusted gross income (MAGI) rules are used in determining eligibility for most of Medicaid's nonelderly populations, including the ACA Medicaid expansion.[19] This change could mean some individuals currently eligible for Medicaid would no longer be found eligible (and vice versa) due to the change in the way income is counted for Medicaid eligibility. For example, the conversion to MAGI might make some children that are currently eligible for Medicaid ineligible because stepparent income is often excluded from current income counting rules but included for MAGI. On the other hand, children currently not eligible might become eligible because MAGI excludes child support income, which is generally included for current income counting rules.[20]

MAGI is defined as the Internal Revenue Code's adjusted gross income (AGI, which reflects a number of deductions, including trade and business deductions, losses from sale of property, and alimony payments) increased (if applicable) by tax-exempt interest and income earned by U.S. citizens or residents living abroad.[21] While the Internal Revenue Service's definition of MAGI excludes non-taxable social security benefits, P.L. 112-56, enacted on

November 21, 2011, changed the definition of income for Medicaid eligibility to include such non-taxable social security benefits.

Under the MAGI counting rules, the state will look at the individual's MAGI, deduct 5%, which the law provides as a standard disregard, and compare that income to the new income standards set by each state in coordination with CMS. See Table A-1 for the new MAGI-based eligibility levels adjusted for the 5% disregard effective January 1, 2014.

The transition to the MAGI income rules has significant implications for the Medicaid eligibility determination process. It represents a major change in terms of the types of information collected (such as what counts as income) and the definition of household (such as the inclusion of the income of a step parent) compared to former Medicaid eligibility rules. These changes necessitate a redesign of the existing Medicaid eligibility and enrollment systems for each state. The system must be integrated with the exchanges as well as with other social programs that serve low-income populations (e.g., the Temporary Assistance for Needy Families [TANF] and the Supplemental Nutrition Assistance Program [SNAP]).

Medicaid Enrollment Trends

Figure 1 shows historical and projected Medicaid enrollment for FY2000 through FY2021 (see Table B-1 for state-by-state Medicaid enrollment for FY2010). The figure shows steady enrollment growth, especially among non-disabled children and adults, punctuated by years of faster enrollment growth in periods immediately after recessions.[22] During periods of economic downturn, state Medicaid programs face program enrollment increases at a faster rate because job and income losses make more people eligible. One study estimated that for every 1% increase in the national unemployment rate, Medicaid enrollment increases by 1 million individuals.[23]

The ACA changes to Medicaid eligibility (including, but not limited to, the ACA Medicaid expansion) are projected to add 8.6 million people to Medicaid in FY2014 and 18.3 million people by FY2021. About 83% of new adult enrollees are projected to be "newly eligible" (i.e., eligible for Medicaid through the ACA Medicaid expansion), while 17% are projected to be individuals who would have been eligible for Medicaid prior to the ACA changes, but were not enrolled.[24]

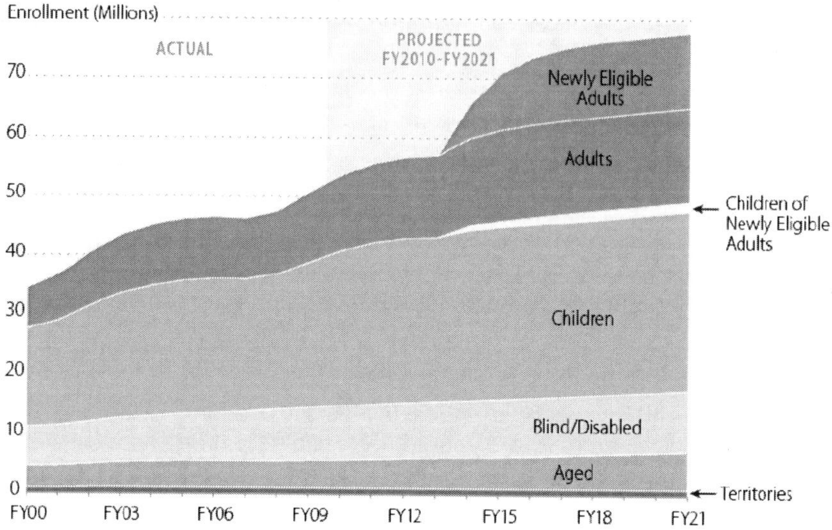

Source: Christopher J. Truffer, John D. Klemm, and Christian J. Wolfe, et al., *2012 Actuarial Report on the Financial Outlook for Medicaid*, Centers for Medicare & Medicaid Services' Office of the Actuary, 2013.

Notes: Enrollment is measured by "person-year equivalents," which is the average enrollment over the course of the year.

For purposes of this figure, "Newly Eligible Adults" are adult enrollees who are newly eligible in 2014 and later as a result of the expanded eligibility criteria in the ACA. "Children of Newly Eligible Adults" are defined here as the dependent children of newly eligible adult enrollees, even if these children were eligible under current criteria. Currently eligible adults who become enrolled as a result of the publicity and outreach efforts associated with the ACA are included with "Adults," and their dependent children are included with "Children" in this figure.

Figure 1. Past and Projected Medicaid Enrollment, by Population; FY2000–FY2021.

Share of Enrollment versus Expenditures, by Population

Different Medicaid enrollment groups have very different service utilization patterns. Larger enrollment groups account for a smaller proportion of the Medicaid expenditures and some smaller enrollment groups are responsible for a larger proportion of Medicaid expenditures. As shown in Figure 2, for FY2011, roughly half of Medicaid enrollees were children without disabilities, who accounted for only about 20% of Medicaid's total benefit spending. The next-largest enrollee group—adults—accounted for about 24% of all enrollees, but only about 15% of benefit expenditures. In contrast, individuals with disabilities represented about 17% of Medicaid enrollees, but accounted for the largest share of Medicaid benefit spending (about 44%). Finally, the elderly represented about 9% of Medicaid enrollees, but about 20% of all benefit spending. While these statistics vary somewhat from year to year and state to state, the patterns described above generally hold true across years.[25]

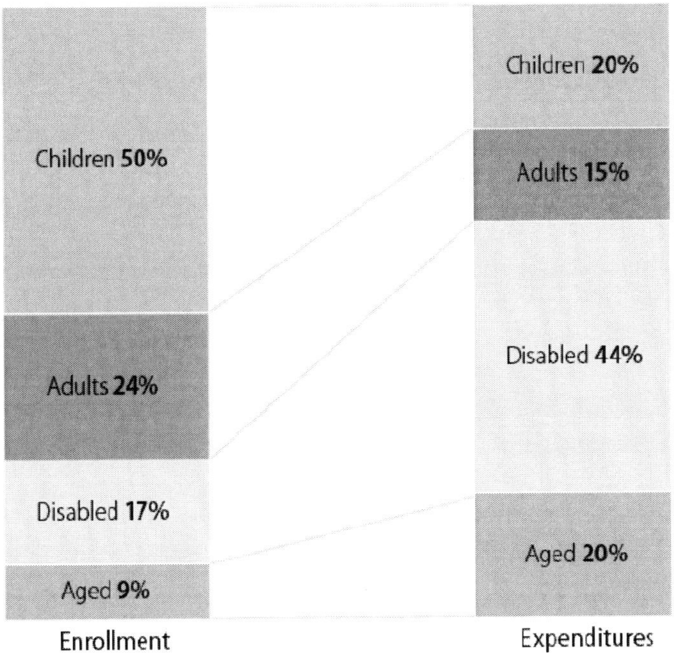

Source: Christopher J. Truffer, John D. Klemm, and Christian J. Wolfe, et al., *2012 Actuarial Report on the Financial Outlook for Medicaid*, Centers for Medicare & Medicaid Services' Office of the Actuary, 2013.

Notes: Totals and components exclude DSH expenditures (i.e., payments to hospitals treating large numbers of low-income patients), territory enrollees and expenditures, and other adjustments.

Figure 2. Estimated Medicaid Enrollment and Expenditures for Benefits, by Enrollment Group as a Share of Total; FY2011.

BENEFITS

Federal law provides two primary benefit packages for state Medicaid programs: (1) traditional benefits and (2) alternative benefit plans (ABPs). Each of these packages is summarized below. In addition, states can use waiver authority (e.g., Section 1115 of the Social Security Act) to tailor benefit packages to specified Medicaid subgroups (see "Medicaid Program Waivers" for more information about Section 1115 waivers).

Traditional Medicaid Benefits

The traditional Medicaid program requires states to cover a wide array of mandatory services (e.g., inpatient hospital care, lab/x-ray services, physician care, nursing facility services for individuals aged 21 and over). In addition, states may provide optional services, some of which are commonly covered (e.g., personal care services for the frail elderly and individuals with disabilities who need long-term services and supports, prescribed drugs, physician-directed clinical services, physical therapy, and prosthetic devices).

States define the specific features of each covered benefit within four broad federal guidelines:

- Each service must be sufficient in "amount, duration, and scope" to reasonably achieve its purpose. States may place appropriate limits on a service based on such criteria as medical necessity.
- Within a state, services available to the various categorically needy groups[26] must be equal in amount, duration, and scope. These requirements are the "comparability" rule.
- With certain exceptions, the amount, duration, and scope of benefits must be the same statewide, referred to as the "statewideness" rule.
- With certain exceptions, enrollees must have "freedom of choice" among health care providers or managed care entities participating in Medicaid.

The breadth of coverage for a given benefit can, and does, vary from state to state, even for mandatory services. For example, states may place different limits on the amount of inpatient hospital services a beneficiary can receive in a year (e.g., up to 15 inpatient days per year in one state versus unlimited inpatient days in another state)—as long as applicable requirements are met regarding comparability; statewideness; and sufficiency of amount, duration, and scope. Exceptions to state limits may be permitted under circumstances defined by the state.

The federal Medicaid statute also delineates special benefits or special rules regarding certain benefits for targeted populations. For example:

- Most Medicaid children under age 21 are entitled to *Early and Periodic Screening, Diagnostic and Treatment (EPSDT) services*. Under EPSDT, children receive well-child visits, immunizations, laboratory tests, and other screening services at regular intervals. In addition, medical care that is necessary to correct or ameliorate identified defects, physical and mental illness, and other conditions must be provided, including some services that states may not otherwise cover in their Medicaid programs.
- *Unauthorized aliens* (i.e., illegal aliens, foreign nationals who are not lawfully present in the United States) are ineligible for Medicaid. Individuals who meet the eligibility requirements for Medicaid but are ineligible due to immigration status may receive Medicaid coverage for emergency conditions (i.e., emergency Medicaid) only, which includes costs associated with emergency labor and delivery for pregnant women and excludes costs for organ transplants.
- Special benefit rules apply to optional *medically needy populations* (for more information about the medically needy see "Eligibility"). States may offer a more restrictive benefit package than is provided to categorically needy populations, but at a minimum, must offer (1) prenatal, delivery, and postpartum services for pregnant women, (2) ambulatory services as defined in the state Medicaid plan for individuals under 18 and those entitled to institutional services, and (3) home health services for individuals entitled to nursing facility care.[27]
- Medicaid law gives states the option to extend *home- and community-based services* (HCBS) to Medicaid enrollees under the HCBS state plan option (Section 1915[i] of the Social Security Act) without requiring a Secretary-approved waiver for this purpose (under Sections 1915[c] or 1115 of the Social Security Act).

Alternative Benefit Plans (ABPs)

Alternative benefit plans (ABPs) are a Medicaid benefit structure that has different requirements than the traditional Medicaid benefits.[28] For example, under ABPs states may waive the "statewideness" and "comparability" requirements that apply under traditional Medicaid. This flexibility permits the state to define populations that will be served and the specific benefit packages that will apply. In general, ABPs may cover fewer benefits than traditional Medicaid, but there are some requirements, such as coverage of EPSDT services, family planning services and supplies, and both emergency and non-emergency transportation to and from providers that might make them more generous than private insurance.

States that choose to implement the ACA Medicaid expansion are required to provide the individuals newly eligible for Medicaid through the expansion Medicaid services through ABPs (with exceptions for selected special-needs subgroups). In addition, states have the option to provide ABP coverage to other subgroups.

ABPs must cover at least the 10 essential health benefits (EHBs) that also apply to the qualified health plans offered in the exchanges.[29] In addition, ABP coverage must comply with the federal requirements for mental health parity,[30] and special rules also apply with regard to prescription drugs, rehabilitative and habilitative services and devices, and preventive care.

Rules regarding how states must design their Medicaid ABPs to meet the ACA requirements have been established through regulation.[31] As a part of the benefit design process, CMS established a policy whereby states can use benefit substitution as a tool to fill in coverage gaps to ensure that all EHBs are represented and/or to align their benefit plans with traditional Medicaid state plan coverage and/or with exchange coverage.[32] This substitution policy has the potential to make Medicaid ABP benefit coverage look very different than the benchmark and benchmark-equivalent benefit coverage that existed prior to ABPs.

Medicaid Benefits by Eligibility Classification

Table 1 provides examples of Medicaid benefits available by selected eligibility classifications. As illustrated, different Medicaid subpopulations may have access to quite varied benefit packages.

Table 1. Examples of Medicaid Benefits, by Eligibility Classification

Eligibility Classification				
Type of Benefit	Traditional Medicaid Populations[a]	Medically Needy	Section 1115 Waivers	Non-Elderly, Non-Pregnant Adults
Mandatory	-Inpatient hospital -Nursing facility care (age 21+) -EPSDT (< age 21) -Physicians -Federally qualified health centers -Family planning -Pregnancy-related services	-Prenatal and delivery services -Ambulatory services (< age 18; individuals entitled to institutional care) -Home health for those entitled to nursing facility care	-Negotiated between the states and the Secretary of HHS	-ABPs
Optional	-Clinic services -Prescribed drugs -Physical, occupational, and speech therapy -Other practitioners -Dental	-Nursing facility care -Clinic services -Physical, occupational, and speech therapy -Other practitioners -Dental	-Negotiated between the states and Secretary of HHS	-For special needs subgroups, option to have same benefits as categorically needy or enroll in an ABP
Traditional Benefits Versus ABPs	Traditional Benefits	Traditional Benefits	Not applicable	ABPs with exceptions

Sources: Title XIX of the Social Security Act and related federal guidance.

Note: With respect to medically needy groups, broader requirements apply if a state has chosen to provide coverage for medically needy individuals in intermediate care facilities for the mentally retarded or in institutions for mental diseases. In these cases, states are required to cover the same services as those which are mandatory for the categorically needy, or alternatively, the care and services described in 7 of the first 24 paragraphs in the federal Medicaid statute defining covered mandatory and optional services.

ABP—Alternative Benefit Plans EPSDT—Early and Periodic Screening, Diagnostic and Treatment services HHS—Health & Human Services

a. Traditional Medicaid populations include the elderly, individuals with disabilities, children, and pregnant women.

Service Delivery Models

Benefits are made available to Medicaid enrollees via two alternative service delivery systems: fee-for-service or managed care. Under the "fee for service" (FFS) delivery system, health care providers are paid by the state Medicaid program for each service provided to a Medicaid enrollee. Under the "managed care" delivery system, Medicaid enrollees get most or all of their services from an organization under contract with the state. States have traditionally used the feefor-service service delivery model for Medicaid, but since the 1990s, the share of Medicaid enrollees covered by the managed care model has increased dramatically. As of July 2011, more than 74% of Medicaid enrollees were covered by some form of managed care.[33]

There are three types of Medicaid managed care:

- **Managed care organizations (MCOs)**—states contract with MCOs to provide a comprehensive package of benefits to certain Medicaid enrollees. States usually pay the MCOs on a capitated basis, which means the states prospectively pay the MCOs a fixed monthly rate per enrollee to provide or arrange for most health care services.
- **Primary care case management (PCCM)**—states contract with primary care providers to provide case management services to Medicaid enrollees. Typically, under PCCM, the primary care provider receives a monthly case management fee per enrollee for coordination of care, but the provider continues to receive FFS payments for the medical care services utilized by Medicaid enrollees.
- **Limited benefit plans**—these plans look like MCOs in that states usually contract with a plan and pay them on a capitated basis. The difference is that limited benefit plans provide only one or two Medicaid benefits (i.e., behavioral health or dental services).

While managed care has largely been used for Medicaid subgroups that do not have chronic health care needs, some states are turning to this type of service delivery system for the elderly and individuals with disabilities.

Medicaid Service Spending

Figure 3 below shows the nationwide distribution of Medicaid expenditures across broad categories of service for FY2012. These data illustrate that roughly one-third of benefit spending is for acute care services, while capitated payments under managed care arrangements account for another third, and LTSS represent slightly more than one-fourth of Medicaid benefit payments. In general, when other sources of insurance/payment are available (including Medicare), Medicaid wraps around that coverage.[34]

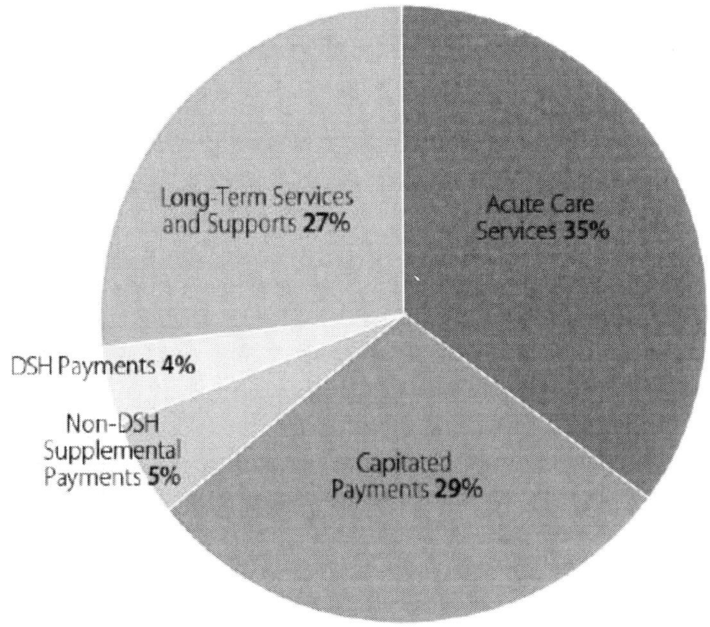

Source: Centers for Medicare & Medicaid Services, CMS-64 Data (base expenditures), FY2012.

Notes: Medical assistance expenditures exclude Medicaid expenditures for administrative activities. DSH stands for "disproportionate share hospital" payments, which are provided in addition to Medicaid payments otherwise received by certain qualifying hospitals.

Figure 3. Medicaid Medical Assistance Payments, by Category; FY2012.

Beneficiary Cost-Sharing

Federal statutes and regulations address the circumstances under which enrollees may share in the costs of Medicaid, both in terms of participation-related cost-sharing (e.g., monthly premiums) and point-of-service cost-sharing (e.g., copayments to providers). States can require certain beneficiaries to share in the cost of Medicaid services, but there are limits on (1) the amounts that states can impose, (2) the beneficiary groups that can be required to pay, and (3) the services for which cost-sharing can be charged.

In general, premiums and enrollment fees are often prohibited. However, premiums may be imposed on enrollees with incomes above 150% of FPL. In state fiscal year (SFY) 2013, 39 states had at least one group able to participate in Medicaid by paying a premium, with a total of 59 different premium programs.[35]

States can impose cost sharing, such as copayments, coinsurance, deductibles, and other similar charges, on most Medicaid-covered benefits, both inpatient and outpatient services, but cost sharing cannot be imposed for emergency services and family planning services and supplies. Some subgroups of beneficiaries are exempt from cost sharing (e.g., children under 18 years of age and pregnant women). The cost-sharing amounts that can be charged vary with income. In SFY2013, 46 states (including the District of Columbia) reported having copayment requirements.[36]

Higher beneficiary cost-sharing is allowed in certain circumstances, and recent ACA regulations modified some of these provisions.[37] For example, for non-emergency care in a hospital emergency department, a maximum $8 payment can be charged to individuals with family income at or below 150% of FPL,[38] and there is no specified limit for individuals with income above 150% of FPL when alternative providers are available.

The aggregate cap on all out-of-pocket cost-sharing is generally up to 5% of monthly or quarterly income.[39]

FINANCING[40]

The federal government and the states jointly finance Medicaid. The federal government reimburses states for a portion (i.e., the federal share) of each state's Medicaid program costs. Because federal Medicaid funding is an open-ended entitlement to states, there is no upper limit or cap on the amount of federal Medicaid funds a state may receive. In FY2012, Medicaid expenditures totaled $431 billion. The federal share totaled $249 billion and the state share was $182 billion.[41]

Federal Share

The federal government's share of most Medicaid expenditures is established by the federal medical assistance percentage (FMAP) rate, which is generally determined annually and varies by state according to each state's per capita income relative to the U.S. per capita income.[42] The formula provides higher FMAP rates, or federal reimbursement rates, to states with lower per capita incomes and lower FMAP rates to states with higher per capita incomes.

FMAP rates have a statutory minimum of 50.00% and a statutory maximum of 83.00%.[43] In FY2014, 15 states have the statutory minimum FMAP rate of 50.00% (Rhode Island is slightly above at 50.11%), and Mississippi has the highest FMAP rate of 73.05% (see Table B-1 for each state's FY2014 FMAP rate).

The FMAP rate is used to reimburse states for the federal share of most Medicaid expenditures, but exceptions to the regular FMAP rate have been made for certain states (e.g., the District of Columbia and the territories), situations (e.g., during economic downturns), populations (e.g., certain women with breast or cervical cancer and individuals in the Qualifying Individuals[44] program), providers (e.g., primary care physicians and Indian Health Service facilities), and services (e.g., family planning and home health services). In addition, the federal share for most Medicaid administrative costs does not vary by state and is generally 50%.

The ACA includes new FMAP exemptions, including the "newly eligible" FMAP rates and the "expansion state" FMAP rates. Under the "newly eligible" FMAP rate, from 2014 through 2016, states receive a 100% FMAP rate for the cost of individuals who are "newly eligible" for Medicaid due to the ACA expansion. This "newly eligible" FMAP rate phases down to 95% in 2017, 94% in 2018, 93% in 2019, and 90% thereafter.[45] The "expansion state" FMAP rate is available for individuals in "expansion states" who were eligible for Medicaid on March 23, 2010, and are in the new eligibility group for nonelderly, nonpregnant adults at or below 133% FPL. The formula[46] used to calculate the "expansion state" FMAP rates is based on a state's regular FMAP rate, so the "expansion state" FMAP rates will vary from state to state until 2019, at which point the "newly eligible" FMAP and the "expansion state" FMAP rates will converge to 93%.

Table 2. FMAP Rates for ACA Medicaid Expansion

	2014	2015	2016	2017	2018	2019	2020+
"Newly eligible" Adults in all States	100%	100%	100%	95%	94%	93%	90%
Certain Individuals in "Expansion states"	75%-92%	80%-93%	85%-95%	86%-93%	90%-93%	93%	90%

Source: Prepared by CRS.

Notes: For the calculation of the "expansion state" FMAP rates, the lower bound is a state with a regular FMAP rate of 50% (which is the statutory minimum), and the upper bound is a state with a regular FMAP rate of 83% (which is the statutory maximum).

While most federal Medicaid funding is provided on an open-ended basis, certain types of federal Medicaid funding are capped. For instance, federal disproportionate share hospital (DSH)[47] funding to states cannot exceed a state-specific annual allotment. Also, Medicaid programs in the territories (i.e., American Samoa, Guam, Northern Mariana Islands, Puerto Rico, and the Virgin Islands) are subject to annual spending caps.

State Share

The federal government provides broad guidelines to states regarding allowable funding sources for the state share (also referred to as the non-federal share) of Medicaid expenditures. However, to a large extent, states are free to determine how to fund their share of Medicaid expenditures. As a result, there is significant variation from state to state in funding sources.

States can use state general funds (i.e., personal income, sales, and corporate income taxes) and "other state funds" (i.e., provider taxes,[48] local government funds, tobacco settlement funds, etc.) to finance the state share of Medicaid.[49] Federal statute[50] allows as much as 60% of the state share to come from local government funding.[51] Federal regulations also stipulate that the state share not be funded with federal funds (Medicaid or otherwise).[52] In SFY2011, on average, 72% of the state share of Medicaid expenditures was financed by state general funds, and the remaining 28% was financed by "other state funds."[53]

A few funding sources have received a great deal of attention over the past couple of decades because states have used these funds in some financing mechanisms designed to maximize the amount of federal Medicaid funds coming to the state. This is referred to as "Medicaid maximization."[54] In general, some states have used "Medicaid maximization" strategies that involve the coordination of fund sources, such as provider taxes and intergovernmental transfers (IGTs),[55] and payment policies, such as DSH and other supplemental payments[56] to draw down federal Medicaid funds without expending many, if any, state general funds.

Expenditures

The cost of Medicaid, like most health expenditures, has generally increased at a rate significantly faster than the overall rate of U.S. economic growth, as measured by Gross Domestic Product (GDP).[57] In the past, much of Medicaid's expenditure growth has been due to federal or state expansions of Medicaid eligibility criteria,[58] but per-enrollee costs for Medicaid have also increased faster than the economy. However, when compared to other forms of health insurance, Medicaid per-enrollee expenditures are relatively low.

One of the major factors impacting Medicaid spending is the economy.[59] Also, state-specific factors, such as policy decisions and demographics, impact Medicaid expenditures and cause Medicaid spending to vary widely from state to state. In 2011 and 2012, Medicaid experienced unusually slow rates of growth, which is the result of improved economic conditions and state efforts to limit the growth of Medicaid expenditures due to the expiration of the temporary increase of the FMAP rate.[60,61]

Figure 4 shows actual Medicaid expenditures from FY1997 to FY2011 and projected Medicaid expenditures from FY2012 through FY2021 (see Table B-1 for state-by-state expenditures for FY2012). These expenditures are broken down by state and federal expenditures. In FY2012, Medicaid spending on services and administrative activities in the 50 states, the District of Columbia, and the territories totaled $431 billion. Medicaid expenditures are estimated to grow to $795 billion in FY2021.[62]

Historically, in a typical year, the average federal share of Medicaid expenditures has been about 57%, which means the average state share is about 43%. However, the federal government's share of Medicaid expenditures is expected to increase with the implementation of the ACA Medicaid expansion because the federal government is funding a vast majority of the cost of the expansion through the "newly eligible" and the "expansion state" FMAP rates. By FY2020, the average federal share of Medicaid is estimated to be 60%.[63]

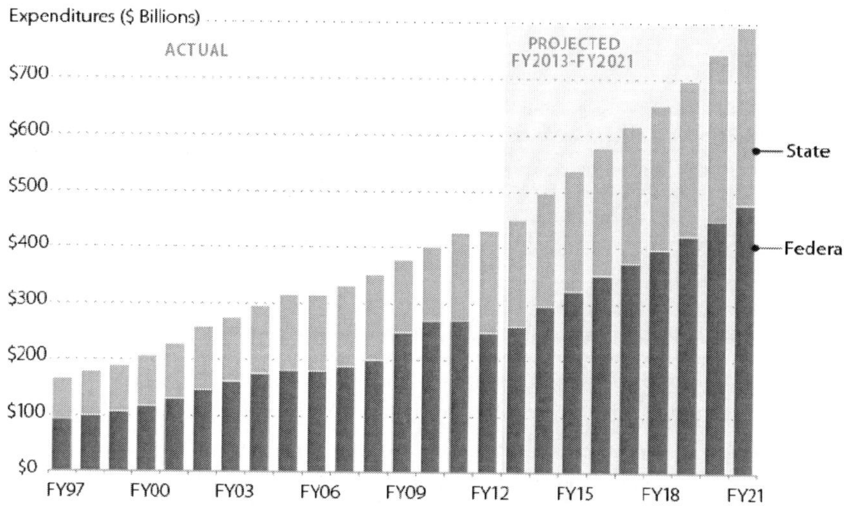

Source: Actual expenditures are from Form CMS-64 Data, and the projected expenditures are from the CMS Office of the Actuary's *2012 Actuary Report on the Financial Outlook for Medicaid.*

Notes: The expenditures shown in this figure include all Medicaid expenditures, which include both administrative and benefit spending.

Figure 4. Federal and State Actual and Projected Medicaid Expenditures; (FY1997 to FY2021; dollars in billions).

PROVIDER PAYMENTS

For the most part, states establish their own payment rates for Medicaid providers. Federal statute requires that these rates be sufficient to enlist enough providers so that covered benefits will be available to Medicaid enrollees at least to the same extent they are available to the general population in the same geographic area.[64]

Low Medicaid physician payment rates in many states and their impact on provider participation have been perennial concerns for policy makers. Still, in recent years, under recessionary budget pressures, many states have reduced Medicaid provider payment rates. Improvements to state finances for

SFY2013 resulted in more states enhancing rather than restricting provider rates for the first time since SFY2009.[65]

The ACA requires that Medicaid payment rates for certain primary care services be raised to what Medicare pays for these services for CY2013 and CY2014. The federal government is picking up the entire cost of that increase in primary care rates (i.e., the difference between Medicare payment rates and the existing Medicaid payment rates as of July 1, 2009) for those two years.

In some cases, states make supplemental payments to Medicaid providers that are separate from and in addition to, the standard payment rates for services rendered to Medicaid enrollees. Often, providers receive supplemental payments in a lump sum. States are permitted to make supplemental payments to providers, but federal regulations specify upper payment limit (UPLs), which prohibit using federal matching funds for Medicaid fee-for-service payments in excess of what would have been paid under Medicare payment principles.[66] The institutions subject to the UPL requirement are hospitals (separated into inpatient services and outpatient services), nursing facilities, intermediate care facilities for the intellectually disabled, and freestanding non-hospital clinics.

Medicaid DSH payments are one type of supplemental payment, and federal statute requires that states make Medicaid DSH payments to hospitals treating large numbers of low-income patients. In FY2012, federal DSH allotments totaled $11.4 billion.[67] The ACA makes aggregate reductions in Medicaid DSH allotments for FY2014 through FY2020. The Middle Class Tax Relief and Job Creation Act of 2012 (P.L. 112-96) and the American Taxpayer Relief Act of 2012 (P.L. 112-240) extended these DSH reductions to FY2021 and FY2022. In FY2023, DSH allotments are scheduled to rebound to the pre-ACA reduced levels.

MEDICAID PROGRAM WAIVERS

The Social Security Act authorizes several waiver and demonstration authorities to provide states with the flexibility to operate their Medicaid programs. Each waiver authority has a distinct purpose and specific requirements. Under the various waiver authorities, states may try new or different approaches to the delivery of health care services or adapt their programs to the special needs of particular geographic areas or groups of Medicaid enrollees. The primary Medicaid waiver authorities include:

- **Section 1115 Research and Demonstration Projects**—Under Section 1115 of the Social Security Act, the Secretary of HHS may waive Medicaid requirements contained in Section 1902 (including, but not limited to, what is known as "freedom of choice" of provider, "comparability" of services, and "statewideness"). States use this waiver authority to change eligibility criteria in order to offer coverage to new groups of people, to provide services that are not otherwise covered, to offer different service packages or a combination of services in different parts of the state, to cap program enrollment, and to implement innovative service delivery systems, among other purposes.
- **Section 1915(b) Managed Care/Freedom of Choice Waivers**—Section 1915(b) of the Social Security Act permits states to establish mandatory managed care programs or otherwise limit enrollees' choice of providers.[68]
- **Section 1915(c) Home- and Community-Based Services Waivers (HCBS)**— Section 1915(c) authorizes the Secretary of HHS to waive certain requirements of Medicaid law allowing states to cover a broad range of HCBS (including services not available under the Medicaid state plan) for certain persons with long-term care needs. Specifically, under Section 1915(c) states can waive rules regarding "statewideness" and "comparability" of services. States may also apply certain income counting rules to persons in HCBS waivers that allow an individual to be eligible for Medicaid who might not otherwise qualify.
- **Section 1915(b) and (c) Waivers**—Section 1915(b) and (c) waivers allow states to provide HCBS to disabled and elderly populations in a managed care setting or within a limited pool of providers. States must apply for each waiver authority concurrently and comply with the individual requirements of each waiver.

States often operate multiple waiver programs with their state plan. Key characteristics of these primary Medicaid waiver authorities compared to state plan requirements are summarized in Table 2. The statutory requirements that may be waived under each type of waiver are different, but all types of waivers are time limited and approvals are subject to reporting and evaluation requirements. In addition, all types of waivers must comply with various financing requirements (i.e., budget neutrality, [69] cost-effectiveness,[70] or cost-neutrality).[71]

Table 3. Key Characteristics of the Primary Medicaid Waiver Authorities Compared to State Plan Requirements

Key Characteristic	Sec. 1115 Research and Demonstration Waivers[a]	Sec. 1915(b) Managed Care/Freedom of Choice Waivers	Sec. 1915(c) Home and Community Based Services (HCBS) Waivers	Sec. 1915(b)/(c) Concurrent Waivers	Medicaid State Plan
Number of Waiversb	73 waivers (in 41 states and DC)	22 waivers (in 18 states)	321 waivers (in 47 states and the District of Columbia)	2 waivers (in 2 states)	N/A
Statutory requirements that may be waived					
"Statewideness"c	X	X	X	X	N/A
"Comparability" of Servicesd	X	X	X	X	N/A
"Freedom of Choice" of Providere	X	X		X	N/A
Income and Resource Rulesf			X	X	N/A
Federal Matching Funds for Costs Not Otherwise Matchable	X	X	X	X	N/A
Evaluations	X	X	X	X	N/A
Duration	5 year initial, renewed for up to 3-year intervals	2 year initial, renewed for up to 2-year intervals	3 year initial, renewed for up to 5-year intervals	Must prepare separate renewal requests	Once approved duration indefinite

Table 3. (Continued)

Key Characteristic	Sec. 1115 Research and Demonstration Waivers[a]	Sec. 1915(b) Managed Care/Freedom of Choice Waivers	Sec. 1915(c) Home and Community Based Services (HCBS) Waivers	Sec. 1915(b)/(c) Concurrent Waivers	Medicaid State Plan
Financing	Budget neutral over the life of the program	Must meet cost-effectiveness test	Must meet cost-neutrality test	Must meet cost-effectiveness neutrality and cost-effectiveness tests	Open-ended mandatory entitlement
Enrollment caps and waiting lists	X		X	X	Individual entitlement

Source: Prepared by CRS based in program rules and regulations.

[a]The number of Section 1115 waivers includes only those under the oversight of CMS's Children and Adults Health Programs Group. This count includes standalone family planning waivers.

[b]Data for number of waivers from lists of operational waivers posted on the CMS website as of 12/4/13.

[c]Waiving the "statewideness" requirement (as permitted under Section 1902[a][1] of the Social Security Act) allows states to target waivers to particular areas of the state where the need is greatest, or where certain types of providers are available, for example.

[d]Waiving "comparability" of services (Section 1902[a][10][B] of the Social Security Act) allows states to target waiver services to particular groups of individuals or to target services on the basis of disease or condition.

[e]Waiving the "freedom of choice" requirement (Section 1902[a][23] of the Social Security Act) allows states to implement managed care delivery systems or otherwise limit choice of provider.

[f]Institutional deeming rules (Section 1902[a][10][C][i][II]) of the Social Security Act) means that income and resources are not deemed to the recipient from a spouse or parent. This allows states to cover medically needy individuals under home and community-based service waivers who would not be eligible for waiver services under the community rules, but would be eligible under institutional rules.

PROGRAM INTEGRITY

Program integrity initiatives are designed to combat fraud, wastc, and abuse in the Medicaid program. Some oversight efforts focus on preventing fraud and abuse through effective program management, while others focus on addressing problems after they occur through investigations, recoveries, and enforcement activities. Areas such as eligibility determination have multiple program integrity initiatives, while other areas, such as managed care, receive comparatively little attention.[72]

Multiple agencies at the federal and state levels are involved in program integrity. The federal agencies are CMS, the Office of the Inspector General for the Department of HHS, the Department of Justice, and the Government Accountability Office. The state agencies involved with program integrity activities include the state Medicaid agencies and the federally required Medicaid Fraud Control Units (MFCUs). Coordination of Medicaid program integrity activities can be a problem because there are so many agencies working on program integrity initiatives and each state develops its own approach to program integrity.

The federal government and states contribute equally to fund most Medicaid activities to combat waste, fraud, and abuse, although for some activities, the federal government provides additional funds through enhanced FMAP rates. As mentioned earlier, all states receive the same FMAP rate for administrative expenditures, including most program integrity activities, which is generally 50%. States receive higher FMAP rates for selected administrative activities such as 90% for the startup of MFCUs and 75% for ongoing MFCU operation.

The ACA included some provisions to increase uniformity among Medicare, Medicaid, and CHIP program integrity activities. For instance, the ACA introduced additional provider screening requirements that are applicable to Medicare, Medicaid, and CHIP. The ACA also created an integrated Medicare and Medicaid data repository to enhance program integrity data sharing to be available to federal and state agencies and law enforcement officials. Moreover, the ACA established a recovery audit contractor (RAC) requirement for Medicaid, under which state Medicaid agencies contract with a RAC to identify and recover overpayments and identify underpayments.

Beyond the ACA requirements, states report implementing a number of new and enhanced Medicaid program integrity activities in SFY2013. For example, 26 states reported implementing or enhancing analytical technologies used to prevent improper payments, 11 states implemented or expanded an enhanced provider screening initiatives, 14 states reported new or enhanced public/private data sharing initiatives, and 18 states reported a wide range of other program integrity efforts or initiatives.[73]

SELECTED ISSUES

Currently, the Medicaid program is dealing with several major issues, which mostly stem from the implementation of the ACA. First, the ACA Medicaid expansion began on January 1, 2014. Since the expansion is optional for states, some are implementing the expansion, some states are still deciding, and other states have chosen not to implement the expansion. Second, the coordination of care for dual-eligible beneficiaries is a focus of federal and state policy makers. Also, a new ACA health insurance annual fee may increase Medicaid expenditures through higher Medicaid MCO rates. Finally, the ACA included a Medicaid MOE provision, which expired on January 1, 2014, for adults but continues until 2019 for children.

ACA Medicaid Expansion

The primary goal of the ACA is to increase access to affordable health insurance for the uninsured and to make health insurance more affordable for individuals who already have such coverage. The ACA Medicaid expansion is one of the major insurance coverage provisions included in the law.

As enacted, beginning in 2014, the ACA Medicaid expansion created a new mandatory Medicaid eligibility group: all adults under age 65 with income up to 133% of FPL (effectively 138% FPL) (see "Eligibility" for more information). The ACA requires most of the individuals covered under the ACA Medicaid expansion to receive ABP coverage (see "Benefits" for more information), and the law provides enhanced federal matching rates for coverage of this new eligibility group (see "Federal Share" for more information).

The ACA provided states with the option to implement the ACA Medicaid expansion earlier than 2014. Between April 1, 2010, and January 1, 2014, states had the option to expand Medicaid to individuals up to 133% of FPL, so long as the state did not extend coverage to (1) individuals with higher income before those with lower incomes or (2) parents unless their children are enrolled in the state plan, a waiver, or in other health coverage. Eight states[74] and the District of Columbia elected to implement the ACA Medicaid expansion early.

Originally, it was assumed that all states would implement the ACA Medicaid expansion in 2014 as required by statute because implementation was required in order for states to receive any federal Medicaid funding. However, on June 28, 2012, the United States Supreme Court issued its decision in *National Federation of Independent Business (NFIB) v. Sebelius*[75] finding that the federal government cannot terminate the federal Medicaid funding a state receives for its current Medicaid program if a state refuses to implement the ACA Medicaid expansion.[76]

State Decisions

Since the federal government cannot terminate current Medicaid federal matching funds if a state refuses to implement the Medicaid expansion required by the ACA, the Supreme Court's ruling in *NFIB* effectively made state participation in the ACA Medicaid expansion voluntary. However, if a state accepts the ACA Medicaid expansion funds, it must abide by the new expansion coverage rules.

CMS informed states that they face no deadline for deciding whether to implement the ACA Medicaid expansion, and according to CMS, states can also discontinue the expansion at any time.[77] If states want to take full advantage of the 100% federal financing for the "newly eligible" enrollees, however, they need to implement the expansion on January 1, 2014. The statute explicitly provides the 100% federal funding for the "newly eligible" enrollees for 2014, 2015, and 2016, rather than for the first three years a state implements the expansion.

As of December 19, 2013, 24 states and the District of Columbia were planning to implement the ACA Medicaid expansion on January 1, 2014, and Michigan is planning to implement the expansion on April 1, 2014.[78] Among the remaining states, 5 are still considering the expansion, and 21 states are not implementing the expansion at this time.[79] Figure 5 shows state decisions about implementing the ACA Medicaid expansion.

While there are some exceptions, most of the states implementing the ACA Medicaid expansion tend to have low rates of uninsured individuals (relative to the national average) and traditionally have provided Medicaid coverage to more nondisabled adults through relatively higher Medicaid income eligibility levels. Also, in general, the states *not* implementing the ACA Medicaid expansion have relatively higher rates of uninsured and traditionally have covered fewer nondisabled adults under Medicaid.[80]

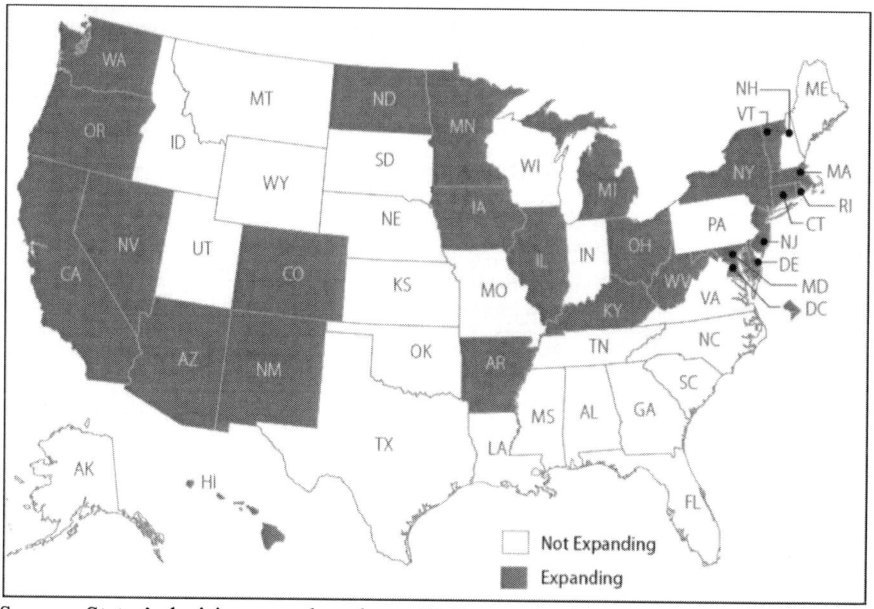

Source: States' decisions are based on CRS's monitoring of state activity through media outlets and state tracking of decisions done by CMS, State Refor(u)m, the Kaiser Family Foundation, the Advisory Board Company, and Avalere.

Notes: All states (except Michigan) are supposed to implement the ACA Medicaid expansion on January 1, 2014. Michigan is planning to implement the expansion on April 1, 2014.

Figure 5. State Decisions Whether to Implement the ACA Medicaid Expansion; As of December 19, 2013.

Premium Assistance Model

Most states implementing the ACA Medicaid expansion are doing so through an expansion of their current Medicaid program. However, some states are using a premium assistance model for their ACA Medicaid expansion, which means Medicaid funding is used to purchase health insurance coverage for the ACA Medicaid expansion population through qualified health plans[81] in the exchanges.

HHS approved Arkansas's waiver to use a premium assistance model for its ACA Medicaid expansion on September 27, 2013, and Iowa's waiver was approved December 10, 2013. Other states (including Florida, Ohio, Pennsylvania, and Tennessee) have expressed interest in the premium assistance model for the ACA Medicaid expansion.[82]

States Not Expanding

States have chosen *not* to implement the ACA Medicaid expansion for various reasons, including not wanting to expand Medicaid because they view the expansion as unaffordable to the state and the Medicaid program as "broken."[83] State decisions *not* to implement the ACA Medicaid expansion could have implications for low-income individuals, large employers with low wage workers, and hospitals.

Low-Income Individuals

Even if a state does *not* implement the ACA Medicaid expansion, some of the individuals that would have been covered by the Medicaid expansion may still gain health insurance coverage under the ACA health insurance coverage provisions. The ACA provides premium tax credits and cost-sharing subsidies to individuals with household income between 100% and 400% of FPL who do not have access to minimum essential coverage.[84] As a result, most uninsured individuals with incomes between 100% and 133% of FPL living in states that decide *not* to implement the ACA Medicaid expansion may become eligible for premium tax credits and cost-sharing subsidies to purchase insurance through the health insurance exchanges. However, most uninsured individuals with incomes under 100% of FPL living in states that decide *not* to implement the ACA Medicaid expansion will likely remain uninsured because these individuals are *not* eligible for premium tax credits or the cost sharing subsidies to purchase health insurance through the exchanges.

Regardless of whether a state decides to implement the ACA Medicaid expansion or not, all states are expected to experience an increase in Medicaid enrollment, due to the "woodwork" effect. This is the term for uninsured individuals who without the expansion are eligible for Medicaid deciding to enroll in Medicaid due to increased media attention and outreach efforts associated with the ACA. The impact of the woodwork effect depends on the percentage of a state's population that is eligible but not enrolled in Medicaid. Nationally, an estimated 7.3 million to 9.0 million uninsured children and adults were eligible but not enrolled in Medicaid prior to the implementation of the expansion.[85]

Large Employers with Low-Wage Workers

Large employers with low-wage workers in states that do *not* implement the ACA Medicaid expansion might have greater exposure to employer penalties included in the ACA when the penalty goes into effect in 2015.[86] The

ACA imposes penalties on "large" employers[87] if at least one of their full-time employees obtains a premium credit through the exchange. Individuals who are not offered employer-sponsored coverage and who are not eligible for Medicaid or other programs may be eligible for premium tax credits for coverage through an exchange. As mentioned above, to receive premium tax credits, individuals must have income of at least 100% and up to 400% of FPL.

In states that do *not* implement the ACA Medicaid expansion, large employers with low income workers could be at greater risk of paying the ACA employer penalty. That is because more low-income workers could qualify for premium tax credits.[88]

Hospitals

Hospitals in states that are *not* expanding Medicaid are concerned because DSH allotments will be reduced by the same across the nation whether or not states implement the expansion. If a state implements the expansion, uncompensated care for hospitals should decline along with the DSH allotments (though not proportionally). However, if a state chooses not to implement the expansion, the demand for uncompensated hospital care is expected to persist but the amount of Medicaid DSH payments hospitals receive to subsidize such care may be reduced.[89] As a result, hospitals have been encouraging states to implement the ACA Medicaid expansion in order to reduce uncompensated care for hospitals. Even though Medicaid provider rates are generally lower than the rates paid by private insurance or Medicare, hospitals are likely better off with payment for a Medicaid patient than no payment for an uninsured patient.

DUAL-ELIGIBLE BENEFICIARIES

In FY2010, there were 9.8 million dual-eligible beneficiaries, who are individuals enrolled in both Medicare and Medicaid,[90] which is almost 15% of Medicaid enrollment. Individuals qualify for Medicare because they are either age 65 or older, or under age 65 and have a disability and have been receiving Social Security Disability Insurance for two years.[91] As mentioned previously, individuals qualify for Medicaid because they meet both the categorical (i.e., are a member of a covered group, such as children, pregnant women, families with dependent children, the elderly, or the disabled) and financial eligibility requirements, which vary by state.

Although commonly addressed as a single population, dual-eligible individuals are a diverse population. While dual-eligible beneficiaries tend to be sicker and poorer than the Medicaid population as a whole, not all dual-eligible beneficiaries are in poor health. Individuals receive different types of Medicaid coverage (i.e., full benefits or financial assistance with Medicare premiums and cost sharing).

There are numerous Medicaid eligibility pathways for dual-eligible beneficiaries,[92] but the two main categories of dual-eligible individuals are full dual-eligible beneficiaries and partial dual-eligible beneficiaries. Full dual-eligible beneficiaries receive full benefits from Medicare, and Medicaid provides them with full benefits in addition to financial assistance with their Medicare premiums and cost sharing. Partial dual-eligible beneficiaries receive full benefits from Medicare and financial assistance from Medicaid for Medicare premiums and cost sharing. In FY2010, there were 7.4 million full duals with Medicaid spending totaling $135.4 billion, while the 2.4 million partial duals had $5.2 billion in Medicaid spending.[93]

Because Medicare and Medicaid are different programs, coordinating care and services for dual-eligible beneficiaries presents challenges. Medicare is a national program administered by CMS, while Medicaid is a federal-state partnership under which each state designs and administers its own version of Medicaid under broad federal rules. Coordination of benefits between these distinct programs is administratively complex. Dual-eligible beneficiaries and their service providers must comply with Medicare and Medicaid program rules and processes, which are not always aligned. In addition, delivery of uncoordinated or poorly coordinated health care and related services can be costly and inefficient, affecting dual-eligible beneficiaries' quality of care and increasing Medicare and Medicaid spending. To reduce spending on dual-eligible beneficiaries and improve the quality of their care, federal and state policy makers are focusing on coordinating care for dual-eligible beneficiaries.[94]

The ACA established the Medicare-Medicaid Coordination Office within CMS in order to improve care coordination for dual-eligible beneficiaries. In addition, the ACA provided CMS the ability to test innovative payment and service delivery models to improve coordination of care and reduce the cost of dual-eligible beneficiaries. With this new authority, CMS is funding demonstration projects to develop approaches to coordinate care for full duals and also to integrate Medicare and Medicaid financing for these individuals.

IMPACT OF ACA HEALTH INSURANCE ANNUAL FEE ON MEDICAID

The ACA imposes an annual fee on certain for-profit health insurers, starting in 2014.[95] The ACA health insurance annual fee applies to Medicaid MCOs with the exception of non-profit insurers incorporated under state law that receive more than 80% of their gross revenues from government programs that target low-income, elderly, or disabled populations (such as CHIP, Medicare, and Medicaid).[96] According to one estimate, approximately 80% of Medicaid enrollees covered by managed care receive coverage from a plan impacted by the ACA fee.[97]

Some insurance plans have informed shareholders and state insurance regulators that they intend to pass on the cost of the fee to businesses and enrollees in the form of higher premiums.[98] Medicaid MCOs do not have the ability to pass the cost of the fee on to enrollees through higher premiums because few Medicaid enrollees pay premiums and when premiums are charged the federal government requires the premiums to be nominal.

A number of state governors caution that the ACA health insurance annual fee will result in higher costs to Medicaid. Federal regulations require that the capitated amounts paid to Medicaid MCOs be "actuarially sound," which means the state must consider MCOs' costs, including health benefits, marketing and administrative expenses, and taxes.[99] For this reason, some states have indicated they are willing to include the cost of the ACA fee in the capitation rates,[100] which will likely increase Medicaid expenditures.

Maintenance of Effort (MOE)

In response to the economic recession (December 2007 through June 2009),[101] Congress enacted the American Recovery and Reinvestment Act of 2009 (ARRA, P.L. 111-5; extended in P.L. 111- 226). ARRA included a temporary increase in FMAP rates. In order to receive federal Medicaid matching funds under ARRA, states were required to maintain the same Medicaid eligibility standards, methodologies, and procedures in effect on July 1, 2008, through June 30, 2011. This provision is referred to as the ARRA MOE requirement.

The ARRA MOE provisions were extended and expanded under the ACA. The ACA MOE provisions were designed to ensure that individuals eligible for Medicaid or CHIP did not lose coverage between the date of enactment of ACA (March 23, 2010) and the implementation of the exchanges. Under the ACA MOE provisions, states were required to maintain their Medicaid programs with the same eligibility standards, methodologies, and procedures until the exchanges were operational. Additionally, the ACA MOE continues for Medicaid-eligible children up to age 19 until September 30, 2019. Failure to comply with the ACA MOE requirements means a state loses all of its federal Medicaid matching funds.

The MOE provision did not prohibit states from cutting Medicaid in other ways, such as by reducing provider rates or by eliminating optional benefits. In addition, states were not prohibited from expanding Medicaid coverage during the MOE period.

The ACA provided an exemption to the MOE requirement for states that had a budget deficit, but only with respect to adults who are non-pregnant and non-disabled adults who are eligible for Medicaid under a state plan or waiver and whose income exceeded 133% of FPL. CMS reports that four states (Hawaii, Illinois, Maine, and Wisconsin) reduced coverage for adults under the ACA MOE exemption authority. Other states, such as Minnesota and Arizona, permitted certain adult populations covered under their Section 1115 waiver programs to end (as permitted through guidance and final regulation) without constituting violation of the ACA MOE requirements.

Under both the ARRA and ACA MOEs, states have not been able to restrict the income eligibility for their Medicaid programs generally speaking from July 1, 2008, through January 1, 2014. With the exception of eligibility standards for children, states now have the ability to reduce the cost of Medicaid through reductions to Medicaid eligibility standards. While state finances are improving, state budgets have not quite recovered from the effects of the recession, and some states welcome an additional budget tool (i.e., reducing Medicaid eligibility thresholds) to reduce the cost of Medicaid.

Eleven states (Illinois, Indiana, Louisiana, Maine, Minnesota, New Mexico, New York, Oklahoma, Rhode Island, Vermont, and Wisconsin) reported plans to tighten eligibility for their adult population groups in 2014.[102] Most of the adults who will lose Medicaid eligibility in these states will be eligible for subsidized coverage through the exchanges.[103] States may be financially better off shifting Medicaid enrollees to the exchanges because the federal government fully funds the cost of premium tax credits and cost-sharing subsidies in the exchanges, whereas states and the federal government share the cost of Medicaid coverage. For the federal government, it is more expensive to cover these individuals through exchanges rather than Medicaid.[104]

Appendix A. State Medicaid and CHIP Income Eligibility Standards

Table A-1 depicts the new MAGI-based eligibility levels for Medicaid beginning on January 1, 2014. The table expresses these standards as a percentage of the federal poverty level (FPL).[105]

Table A-1. Selected State Medicaid MAGI Income Eligibility Standards Expressed as a Percentage of the Federal Poverty Level Effective January 1, 2014

	Children				Adults	
State	Ages 0-1[a]	Ages 1-5[a]	Ages 6-18[a]	Pregnant Women	Parents[b]	Other Adults
Alabama	141%	141%	141%	141%	13%	0
Alaskac	203%	203%	203%	200%	129%	0%d
Arizona	147%	141%	133%	156%	133%	133%
Arkansas	211%	211%	211%	209%	133%	133%
California	261%	261%	261%	208%	133%	133%
Colorado	142%	142%	142%	195%	133%	133%
Connecticut	196%	196%	196%	258%	196%	133%
Delaware	209%	142%	133%	209%	133%	133%
District of Columbia	319%	319%	319%	319%	216%	210%
Florida	206%	140%	133%	191%	31%	0%d
Georgia	205%	149%	133%	220%	36%	0%
Hawaiic	308%	308%	308%	191%	133%	133%
Idaho	141%	141%	133%	133%	24%e	f
Illinois	142%	142%	142%	208%	133%	133%
Indiana	208%	158%	158%	208%	20%e	f
Iowa	375%	167%	167%	375%	133%	133%
Kansas	166%	149%	133%	166%	33%	0%
Kentucky	195%	159%	159%	195%	133%	133%
Louisiana	212%	212%	212%	209%	19%e	f
Maine	191%	157%	157%	209%	100%	d,f
Maryland	317%	317%	317%	259%	133%	133%
Massachusetts	200%	150%	150%	200%	133%	133%d
Michigan	195%	160%	160%	195%	133%	133%
Minnesota	283%	275%	275%	278%	200%	200%
Mississippi	194%	143%	133%	194%	24%	0%
Missouri	205%	150%	150%	205%	20%e	f

State	Ages 0-1[a]	Children Ages 1-5[a]	Ages 6-18[a]	Pregnant Women	Adults Parents[b]	Other Adults
Montana	159%	143%	143%	159%	48%	f
Nebraska	213%	213%	213%	194%	63%	0%
Nevada	159%	159%	133%	159%	133%	133%
New Hampshire	318%	318%	318%	196%	70%	0%
New Jersey	194%	142%	142%	194%	133%	133%
New Mexico	300%	300%	240%	250%	133%	133%
New York	218%	149%	149%	218%	133%	133%[d]
North Carolina	210%	210%	133%	196%	46%	0%d
North Dakota	147%	147%	133%	147%	133%	133%
Ohio	206%	206%	206%	200%	133%	133%
Oklahoma	205%	205%	205%	133%	43%e	f
Oregon	185%	133%	133%	185%	133%	133%
Pennsylvania	215%	157%	133%	215%	33%	0%d
Rhode Island	261%	261%	261%	190%	133%	133%
South Carolina	208%	208%	208%	194%	62%	0%
South Dakota	182%	182%	182%	133%	54%	0%
Tennessee	195%	142%	133%	195%	106%	0%
Texas	198%	144%	133%	198%	15%	0%
Utah	139%	139%	133%	139%	46%e	f
Vermont	313%	313%	313%	208%	133%	133%
Virginia	143%	143%	143%	143%	49%	0%
Washington	207%	207%	207%	193%	133%	133%
West Virginia	158%	141%	133%	158%	133%	133%
Wisconsin	301%	186%	151%	301%	95%e	95%
Wyoming	154%	154%	133%	154%	57%	0%

Source: Centers for Medicare and Medicaid Services. Eligibility levels in effect based on information current as of September 30, 2013, provided to CMS by states either for purposes of FFM programming of state-specific Medicaid/CHIP rules, through state plan amendments, or by direct request from CMS. These levels are subject to change.

Notes: For these eligibility groups, an individual's income, computed based on the new modified adjusted gross income (MAGI)-based income rules and adjusted by a 5% disregard, is compared to the income standards identified in this table to determine if they are income eligible for Medicaid or CHIP. Other eligibility criteria also apply, for example, with respect to citizenship, immigration status and residency. Note that this table reflects the principal but not all MAGI coverage groups.

[a]These eligibility standards include CHIP-funded Medicaid expansions.

[b]In states that use dollar amounts rather than percentages of the federal poverty level (FPL) for 2013 to determine eligibility for parents, CMS has converted those amounts to a percent of the FPL and selected the highest percentage to reflect the eligibility level for the group. In addition, for states that are adopting the Medicaid expansion, CMS has indicated the upper income limit for parents will also be 133% of the FPL, since parents can be eligible for coverage under the new ACA Medicaid expansion group. The actual dollar standards that states will use to determine eligibility are quoted in the monthly income tables available at http://www.medicaid.gov/AffordableCareAct/Medicaid-Moving-Forward-2014/Medicaid-and-CHIP-Eligibility-Levels/medicaid-chip-eligibility-levels.html.

[c]The dollar values that represent the FPLs in Alaska and Hawaii are higher than for the contiguous 48 states. For example, as of 2013, 100% of the FPL for a family of four is equal to $29,440 in Alaska and $27,090 in Hawaii, compared to $23,550 in the other 48 states.

[d]The state covers some 19 and 20 year olds—AK (129%), FL (31%), ME (156%), MA (150%), NY (150%), NC (46%), and PA (33%).

[e]Reflects parent coverage under the Medicaid state plan. The state has some additional coverage above state plan eligibility standards through a section 1115 demonstration or a pending demonstration proposal. The demonstration includes limitations on eligibility and/or benefits, is not offered to all residents of the state, and/or includes an enrollment cap.

[f]The state has a Section 1115 demonstration or a pending demonstration proposal that provides Medicaid coverage to some low-income adults. The demonstration includes limitations on eligibility and/or benefits, is not offered to all residents of the states, and/or includes an enrollment cap.

CMS worked with states to "convert" their Medicaid income eligibility levels to be based on MAGI as required by the ACA. This table provides the Medicaid MAGI income eligibility levels by FPL for the key groups—children, pregnant women, parents/caretaker relatives and other adults—whose eligibility will be MAGI-based beginning in 2014.

APPENDIX B. STATE-BY-STATE MEDICAID DATA

Table B-1 provides the most recent available data for state-by-state Medicaid enrollment, expenditures (including both the federal and state shares), and FMAP rates.

Table B-1. State-by-State Medicaid Enrollment, Expenditures, and FMAP Rates

		FY2012 Medicaid Expenditures[a] ($ in millions)			
State	FY2010 Enrollment[b] (in thousands)	State	Federal	Total	FY2014 FMAP Rates
Alabama	1,016	$1,613	$3,589	$5,202	68.12
Alaska	126	$587	$854	$1,441	50.00
Arizona	1,531	$2,528	$5,639	$8,167	67.23
Arkansas	699	$1,288	$3,074	$4,362	70.10
California	11,335	$25,749	$27,522	$53,271	50.00
Coloradoc	632	$2,428	$2,488	$4,916	50.00
Connecticut	712	$3,331	$3,366	$6,696	50.00
Delaware	225	$707	$866	$1,573	55.31
District of Columbia	213	$681	$1,544	$2,224	70.00
Florida	3,703	$8,112	$10,535	$18,647	58.79
Georgia	1,870	$2,976	$5,819	$8,795	65.93

Table B-1. (Continued)

		FY2012 Medicaid Expenditures[a] ($ in millions)			
	FY2010 Enrollment[b] (in thousands)	State	Federal	Total	FY2014 FMAP Rates
Hawaii	261	$749	$763	$1,512	51.85
Idahoc	223	$466	$1,050	$1,516	71.64
Illinois	2,780	$6,891	$7,105	$13,995	50.00
Indiana	1,174	$2,627	$5,264	$7,891	66.92
Iowa	555	$1,384	$2,190	$3,574	57.93
Kansas	394	$1,204	$1,631	$2,834	56.91
Kentucky	907	$1,665	$4,094	$5,759	69.83
Louisiana	1,177	$2,277	$5,077	$7,354	60.98
Mainec	352	$913	$1,652	$2,565	61.55
Maryland	952	$3,907	$3,998	$7,904	50.00
Massachusetts	1,654	$6,595	$6,731	$13,326	50.00
Michigan	2,257	$4,381	$8,560	$12,941	66.32
Minnesota	936	$4,460	$4,544	$9,004	50.00
Mississippi	772	$1,181	$3,438	$4,618	73.05
Missouric	1,033	$3,261	$5,743	$9,004	62.03
Montana	133	$336	$695	$1,031	66.33
Nebraska	250	$768	$1,024	$1,792	54.74
Nevada	340	$787	$1,045	$1,832	63.10
New Hampshire	167	$614	$637	$1,251	50.00
New Jersey	1,026	$5,404	$5,567	$10,971	50.00
New Mexico	576	$1,063	$2,541	$3,604	69.20
New York	5,570	$26,305	$26,769	$53,074	50.00
North Carolina	1,876	$4,458	$8,418	$12,876	65.78
North Dakota	82	$342	$446	$788	50.00
Ohio	2,246	$6,058	$10,768	$16,826	63.02
Oklahoma	829	$1,639	$3,005	$4,644	64.02
Oregon	644	$1,819	$3,103	$4,922	63.14
Pennsylvania	2,417	$9,466	$11,684	$21,150	53.52
Rhode Island	205	$912	$1,032	$1,944	50.11
South Carolina	909	$1,434	$3,381	$4,815	70.57
South Dakota	131	$293	$492	$786	53.54
Tennessee	1,502	$3,115	$6,135	$9,250	65.29
Texas	4,844	$11,998	$16,936	$28,934	58.69
Utah	352	$593	$1,410	$2,003	70.34
Vermont	196	$570	$792	$1,362	55.11
Virginia	1,007	$3,511	$3,579	$7,089	50.00
Washington	1,353	$3,949	$4,171	$8,120	50.00
West Virginia	430	$810	$2,121	$2,931	71.09
Wisconsinc	1,139	$2,898	$4,566	$7,464	59.06
Wyoming	87	$270	$296	$566	50.00
National Total	65,804	$181,370	$247,748	$429,118	

Source: Medicaid and CHIP Payment and Access Commission, *Report to Congress on Medicaid and CHIP*, March 2013; Centers for Medicare & Medicaid Services, CMS-64 data; Department of Health and Human Services, "Federal Financial Participation in State Assistance Expenditures; Federal Matching Shares for Medicaid, the Children's Health Insurance Program, and Aid to Needy Aged, Blind, or Disabled Persons for October 1, 2013 Through September 30, 2014," 77 *Federal Register* 71420, November 30, 2012.

Notes: May not sum to totals due to rounding.

[a]Medicaid expenditures include benefit and administrative expenditures but exclude expenditures in the territories and spending for State Medicaid Fraud Control Units, Medicaid survey and certification of nursing and intermediate care facilities, and the Vaccines for Children program.

[b]Enrollment numbers generally include individuals ever enrolled in Medicaid-financed coverage during the year, even if for a single month. Numbers exclude enrollees in the territories.

[c]Enrollment data for FY2010 was not available for Colorado, Idaho, Maine, Missouri, and Wisconsin, and this table show FY2009 for these states.

End Notes

[1] This enrollment figure is measured according to "person-year equivalents," which represents the average program enrollment over the course of a year, and differs from "ever enrolled" counts which measure the number of people covered by Medicaid for any period of time during the year. (Office of the Actuary [OACT], Centers for Medicare and Medicaid Services, U.S. Department of Health and Human Services, *National Health Expenditure Projections 2012- 2022: Forecast Summary,* 2013.)

[2] Centers for Medicare & Medicaid Services, CMS-64 data.

[3] The health care safety net is defined as those organizations and programs, in both the public and private sectors, with a legal obligation or a commitment to provide direct health care services to uninsured and underinsured populations.

[4] Calculation based on data from Medicaid and CHIP Payment and Access Commission (MACPAC), *Overview of Medicaid and CHIP,* January 2013.

[5] CRS analysis of National Health Expenditure Account (NHEA) data obtained from the Centers for Medicare and Medicaid Services (CMS), Office of the Actuary, December 16, 2012; MACPAC, *Overview of Medicaid and CHIP*, January 2013.

[6] MACPAC, *Report to the Congress on Medicaid and CHIP*, June 2013.

[7] Micah Hartman, Anne B. Martin, and Joseph Benson, et al., "National Health Spending in 2011: Overall Growth Remains Low, But Some Payers and Services Show Signs of Acceleration," *Health Affairs*, vol. 32, no. 1 (2013), pp. 87-99.

[8] The five territories are American Samoa, Guam, the Commonwealth of the Northern Mariana Islands, Puerto Rico, and the Virgin Islands.

[9] Medicaid is an entitlement for both states and individuals. The Medicaid entitlement to states ensures that, so long as states operate their programs within the federal requirements, states are entitled to federal Medicaid matching funds. Medicaid is also an individual entitlement, which means that anyone eligible and enrolled in Medicaid under his or her state's eligibility standards is guaranteed Medicaid coverage.

[10] The state plan outlines Medicaid eligibility standards, provider requirements, payment methods, and health benefit packages among other program design criteria. Although this

report describes federal Medicaid requirements, a number of these requirements can be waived, with approval from the Secretary of Health and Human Services (HHS), as discussed in the subsection on waivers.

[11] See "Benefits" section for a discussion of these benefits.

[12] For more information see CRS Report R42978, *Comparing Medicaid and Exchanges: Benefits and Costs for Individuals and Families*.

[13] Exchanges were established under the ACA as market places where certain individuals and businesses can purchase private health insurance. For more information about the exchanges, see CRS Report R42663, *Health Insurance Exchanges Under the Patient Protection and Affordable Care Act (ACA)*, by Bernadette Fernandez and Annie L. Mach.

[14] For more information, see CRS Report R42978, *Comparing Medicaid and Exchanges: Benefits and Costs for Individuals and Families*.

[15] Some groups, such as young people under the age of 26 who have aged out of foster care, are eligible for Medicaid coverage without regard to the youths' income and assets.

[16] The poverty guidelines (also referred to as the federal poverty level) are a version of the federal poverty measure. They are issued each year in the *Federal Register* by the Department of Health and Human Services (HHS). The guidelines are a simplification of the poverty thresholds for use for administrative purposes—for instance, determining financial eligibility for certain federal programs.

[17] For these groups, states are required to allow individuals to spend down to the medically needy income standard by incurring and paying medical expenses.

[18] 42 CFR §435.603(d)(4).

[19] Under ACA, certain groups are exempt from income eligibility determinations for Medicaid based on MAGI. Prior law's income determination rules under Medicaid will continue to be used for determining eligibility for the following groups: (1) individuals who are eligible for Medicaid through another federal or state assistance program (e.g., foster care children and individuals receiving SSI), (2) the elderly, (3) certain disabled individuals who qualify for Medicaid on the basis of being blind or disabled without regard to whether the individual is eligible for SSI, (4) the medically needy, and (5) enrollees in a Medicare Savings Program (e.g., Qualified Medicare Beneficiaries for whom Medicaid pays the Medicare premiums or coinsurance and deductibles). In addition, MAGI does not affect eligibility determinations through Express Lane enrollment (to determine whether a child has met Medicaid or CHIP eligibility requirements), for Medicare prescription drug low-income subsidies, or for determinations of eligibility for Medicaid long-term services and supports.

[20] John L. Czajka, *Translating Modified Adjusted Gross Income (MAGI) to Current Monthly Income*, State Health Access Reform Evaluation, May 2013.

[21] For more information, see CRS Report R41997, *Definition of Income for Certain Medicaid Provisions and Premium Credits in ACA*.

[22] According to the National Bureau of Economic Analysis, the United States was in recession from March 2001 through November 2001 and December 2007 through June of 2009.

[23] John Holahan and A. Bowen Garrett, *Rising Unemployment, Medicaid and the Uninsured*, Kaiser Commission on Medicaid and the Uninsured, Publication #7850, January 2009.

[24] Office of the Actuary (OACT), Centers for Medicare & Medicaid Services, U.S. Department of Health & Human Services, *2012 Actuarial Report on the Financial Outlook for Medicaid*, 2013.

[25] Office of the Actuary (OACT), Centers for Medicare & Medicaid Services, U.S. Department of Health & Human Services, *2012 Actuarial Report on the Financial Outlook for Medicaid*, 2013.

[26] Categorically needy groups include families with children, the elderly, persons with disabilities, and certain other pregnant women and children who meet former AFDC- and SSI-related financial standards, or have income below specified percentages of the FPL. Beginning in 2014, or earlier at state option, this classification will also include non-elderly, non-pregnant adults.

[27] Broader requirements apply if a state has chosen to provide coverage for medically needy persons in institutions for mental disease and intermediate care facilities for the mentally retarded. In these cases, states are required to cover the same services as those which are mandatory for the categorically needy, or alternatively, the care and services described in 7 of the first 24 paragraphs in the federal Medicaid statute defining covered mandatory and optional services.

[28] Prior to the ACA, ABPs were referred to as benchmark and benchmark-equivalent benefit packages (as per the Deficit Reduction Act of 2005, P.L. 109-171). Pre-ACA Benchmark coverage included one of the four benchmark options: (1) the standard Blue Cross/Blue Shield preferred provider option offered through the Federal Employees Health Benefit program; (2) State employee coverage that is offered and generally available to state employees; (3) commercial HMO with the largest insured commercial non-Medicaid enrollment in the state; and/or (4) Secretary-approved coverage, a benefit package the Secretary has determined to provide coverage appropriate to meet the needs of the population. Pre-ACA Benchmark-equivalent coverage was required to have the same aggregate actuarial value as one of the benchmark plans and was also required to include (1) inpatient and outpatient hospital services; (2) physician services; (3) lab and x-ray services; (4) emergency care; (5) well-child care, including immunizations; (6) prescribed drugs; (7) mental health services; and (8) other appropriate preventive care (designated by the Secretary). Such coverage was also required include at least 75% of the actuarial value of coverage under the applicable ABP for vision care and hearing services (if any).

[29] The 10 essential health benefits required under the ACA include (1) ambulatory patient services, (2) emergency services, (3) hospitalization, (4) maternity and newborn care, (5) mental health and substance use disorder services (including behavioral health treatment), (6) prescribed drugs, (7) rehabilitative and habilitative services and devices, (8) laboratory services, (9) preventive and wellness services and chronic disease management, and (10) pediatric services, including oral and vision care.

[30] Health insurance coverage for mental illness had historically been less generous than that for other physical illnesses. Mental health parity is a response to this disparity in insurance coverage, and generally refers to the concept that health insurance coverage for mental health services should be offered on par with covered medical and surgical benefits. For more information about mental health parity, see CRS Report R41249, *Mental Health Parity and the Patient Protection and Affordable Care Act of 2010*, by Amanda K. Sarata.

[31] Centers for Medicare and Medicaid Services (CMS), "Medicaid and Health Insurance Programs: Essential Health Benefits in Alternative Benefit Plans, Eligibility Notices, Fair Hearing and Appeal Processes, and Premiums and Cost Sharing; Exchanges: Eligibility and Enrollment," Final Rule, 78 *Federal Register*, July 15, 2013.

[32] For a discussion of the substitution process, see CRS Report R43328, *Medicaid Coverage of Long-Term Services and Supports*, by Kirsten J. Colello.

[33] Centers for Medicare & Medicaid Services, *Medicaid Managed Care Enrollment Report*, November 2012.

[34] For related details, see Federal regulations at 42 CFR 433.135, 433.138, and 433.152.

[35] Vernon K. Smith, Robin Rudowitz, and Laura Snyder, *Medicaid in a Historic Time of Transformation: Results from a 50-State Medicaid Budget Survey for State Fiscal Years 2013 and 2014*, Kaiser Commission on Medicaid and the Uninsured, October 2013

[36] Vernon K. Smith, Robin Rudowitz, and Laura Snyder, *Medicaid in a Historic Time of Transformation: Results from a 50-State Medicaid Budget Survey for State Fiscal Years 2013 and 2014*, Kaiser Commission on Medicaid and the Uninsured, October 2013

[37] Department of Health and Human Services, Centers for Medicare and Medicaid Services, Essential Health Benefits in Alternative Benefit Packages, Eligibility Notices, Fair Hearing and Appeal Processes, and Premiums and Cost Sharing; Exchanges; Eligibility and Enrollment; Final rule, *Federal Register*, Vol. 78, No. 135, July 15, 2013.

[38] Beginning October 1, 2015, such cost-sharing must be increased by the percentage increase in the medical care component of the CPI-U for the period of September to September of the preceding calendar year, rounded to the next higher 5-cent increment.

[39] Section 1916A of the Social Security Act.

[40] For more information about Medicaid financing and expenditures, see CRS Report R42640, *Medicaid Financing and Expenditures*, by Alison Mitchell.

[41] Centers for Medicare & Medicaid Services, CMS-64 data.

[42] For more detail about the FMAP rate, see CRS Report R42941, *Medicaid's Federal Medical Assistance Percentage (FMAP), FY2014*, by Alison Mitchell and Evelyne P. Baumrucker.

[43] Section 1905(b) of the Social Security Act.

[44] States are required to pay Medicare Part B premiums for Medicare beneficiaries with income between 120% and 135% FPL and limited assets (referred to as "qualifying individuals"), up to a specified dollar allotment.

[45] The "newly eligible" FMAP rates are available for these specific years, regardless of whether a state implements the ACA Medicaid expansion in 2014 or a later year.

[46] Expansion state FMAP formula = [regular FMAP + (newly eligible FMAP – regular FMAP) * transition percentage equal to 50% in CY2014, 60% in CY2015, 70% in CY2016, 80% in CY2017, 90% in CY2018, and 100% in CY2019+].

[47] For more information about Medicaid DSH payments, see CRS Report R42865, *Medicaid Disproportionate Share Hospital Payments*, by Alison Mitchell.

[48] States are able to use revenues from health care provider taxes to help finance their share of Medicaid expenditures as long as the provider tax is broad-based and uniform. Also, states are not allowed to hold the providers harmless for the cost of the provider tax (i.e., they cannot guarantee that providers receive their money back). In addition, provider tax revenue is prohibited from exceeding 25% of the state share of Medicaid expenditures. For more information about provider taxes, see CRS Report RS22843, *Medicaid Provider Taxes*, by Alison Mitchell.

[49] National Association of State Budget Officers, *State Expenditure Report: Examining Fiscal 2011-2013 State Spending*, 2013.

[50] Section 1902(a)(2) of the Social Security Act.

[51] The federal statute allows for the significant use of local funds in financing Medicaid because local governments financed a significant amount of the health care services provided to low-income individuals prior to the enactment of Medicaid. (Medicaid and CHIP Payment and Access Commission, *Report to the Congress on Medicaid and CHIP*, March 2012.)

[52] 42 C.F.R. 433.51(c).

[53] National Association of State Budget Officers, *State Expenditure Report: Examining Fiscal 2011-2013 State Spending*, 2013.

[54] National Health Policy Forum at The George Washington University, *The Basics: Medicaid Financing*, February 4, 2011; U.S. Government Accountability Office, *Medicaid Financing: Long-Standing Concerns about Inappropriate State Arrangements Support Need for Improved Federal Oversight*, testimony of Marjorie Kanof before U.S. Congress, House of Representatives, Committee on Oversight and Government Reform, GAO-08-255T, November 1, 2007; Andy Schneider and David Rousseau, *The Medicaid Resource Book*, The Kaiser Commission on Medicaid and the Uninsured, Publication Number 2236, January 17, 2003; Teresa A. Coughlin and Stephen Zuckerman, *States' Use of Medicaid Maximization Strategies to Tap Federal Revenues: Program Implications and Consequences*, The Urban Institute, June 2002.

[55] IGTs are transfers of public funds between government entities, such as from counties to states or between state agencies. This financing mechanism is commonly used to enable states and local governments to carry out shared functions.

[56] Supplemental payments are Medicaid payments made to providers that are separate from and in addition to the standard payment rates for services rendered to Medicaid enrollees. Often, providers receive supplemental payments in a lump sum.

[57] Christopher J. Truffer, John D. Klemm, and Christian J. Wolfe, et al., 2012 Actuarial Report on the Financial Outlook for Medicaid, Centers for Medicare & Medicaid Services' Office of the Actuary, 2013.

[58] Rachel Garfield, Lisa Clemans-Cope, and Emily Lawton, et al., *Enrollment-Driven Expenditure Growth: Medicaid Spending during the Economic Downturn, FFY2007-2010*, Kaiser Commission on Medicaid and the Uninsured, Publication #8309, May 2012.

[59] Christopher J. Truffer, John D. Klemm, and Christian J. Wolfe, et al., 2012 Actuarial Report on the Financial Outlook for Medicaid, Centers for Medicare & Medicaid Services' Office of the Actuary, 2013.

[60] For FY2009 through FY2011, the federal share of Medicaid expenditures was higher than usual due to the temporary FMAP increase provided to states from October 1, 2008, through June 30, 2011. The temporary FMAP increase was originally provided through the American Recovery and Reinvestment Act of 2009 (P.L. 111-5) and extended through P.L. 111-226.

[61] Christopher J. Truffer, John D. Klemm, and Christian J. Wolfe, et al., 2012 Actuarial Report on the Financial Outlook for Medicaid, Centers for Medicare & Medicaid Services' Office of the Actuary, 2013; Anne B. Martin, Micah Hartman, and Lekha Whittle, "National Health Spending in 2012: Rate of Health Spending Growth Remained Low for the Fourth Consecutive Year," *Health Affairs*, vol. 33, no. 1 (January 2014).

[62] U.S. Department of Health and Human Services, Centers for Medicare and Medicaid Services, Form CMS-64 data, April 16, 2012; Christopher J. Truffer, John D. Klemm, and Christian J. Wolfe, et al., *2012 Actuarial Report on the Financial Outlook for Medicaid*, Centers for Medicare & Medicaid Services' Office of the Actuary, 2013.

[63] Congressional Budget Office, *An Overview of the Medicaid Program*, September 18, 2013; Christopher J. Truffer, John D. Klemm, and Christian J. Wolfe, et al., *2012 Actuarial Report on the Financial Outlook for Medicaid*, Centers for Medicare & Medicaid Services' Office of the Actuary, 2013.

[64] Section 1902(a)(30)(A) of the Social Security Act.

[65] Vernon K. Smith, Robin Rudowitz, and Laura Snyder, *Medicaid in a Historic Time of Transformation: Results from a 50-State Medicaid Budget Survey for State Fiscal Years 2013 and 2014*, Kaiser Commission on Medicaid and the Uninsured, October 2013; Vernon K. Smith, Robin Rudowitz, and Laura Snyder, *Medicaid Today; Preparing for Tomorrow A*

Look at Medicaid Spending, Enrollment and Policy Trends: Results from a 50-State Medicaid Budget Survey for State Fiscal Years 2012 and 2013, Kaiser Commission on Medicaid and the Uninsured, October 2012; and Vernon K. Smith, Robin Rudowitz, and Laura Snyder, *Moving Ahead Amid Fiscal Challenges: A Look at Medicaid Spending, Coverage and Policy Trends, Results from a 50-State Medicaid Budget Survey for State Fiscal Years 2011 and 2012*, Kaiser Commission on Medicaid and the Uninsured, October 2011.

[66] In practice, the UPL rules simply ensure that Medicaid does not pay a class of providers in the aggregate more than Medicare would have paid for the same or comparable services delivered by those same institutions. (Medicaid and CHIP Payment and Access Commission, *Medicaid UPL Supplemental Payments*, November 2012.)

[67] DSH allotments are different from DSH payments. Allotments reflect the maximum amount of federal DSH funding available to states, and DSH payments are the amounts paid to hospitals. Each state receives an annual DSH allotment, which is the maximum amount of federal matching funds that each state is permitted to claim for Medicaid DSH payments. For more information about Medicaid DSH payments, see CRS Report R42865, *Medicaid Disproportionate Share Hospital Payments*, by Alison Mitchell.

[68] There are four types of authorities under Section 1915(b) that states may request: (b)(1) allows states to require Medicaid beneficiaries to enroll in managed care; (b)(2) allows states to designate a "central broker" to assist Medicaid beneficiaries in choosing among competing health care plans; (b)(3) allows states to use cost savings made possible through the recipients' use of more cost-effective medical care to provide additional services; and (b)(4) allows states to limit the beneficiaries' choice of providers (except in emergency situations, for recipients residing in a long term care facility, and with respect to family planning services).

[69] Budget neutrality means that the estimated spending under the waiver cannot exceed the estimated cost of the state's Medicaid program without the waiver.

[70] Cost effectiveness means the cost of payments under managed care cannot exceed the cost of fee-for-service absent the waiver.

[71] Under the cost-neutrality test, expenditures under the waiver may not exceed the cost of institutional care that would have been provided to waiver recipients absent the waiver.

[72] Medicaid and CHIP Payment and Access Commission, *Report to Congress on Medicaid and CHIP*, June 2013.

[73] Vernon K. Smith, Robin Rudowitz, and Laura Snyder, *Medicaid in a Historic Time of Transformation: Results from a 50-State Medicaid Budget Survey for State Fiscal Years 2013 and 2014*, Kaiser Commission on Medicaid and the Uninsured, October 2013.

[74] The eight states that implemented the ACA Medicaid expansion early were California, Colorado, Connecticut, Illinois, Minnesota, New Jersey, Ohio, and Washington.

[75] 132 S. Ct. 2566 (2012).

[76] For a discussion of the Supreme Court's decision on the Medicaid expansion, see CRS Report R42367, *Medicaid and Federal Grant Conditions After NFIB v. Sebelius: Constitutional Issues and Analysis*, by Kenneth R. Thomas.

[77] Centers for Medicare & Medicaid Services, *Frequently Asked Questions on the Exchanges, Market Reforms and Medicaid*, December 10, 2012.

[78] The Medicaid expansion for Iowa and Michigan is subject to CMS approval of those states' 1115 Waiver applications. (CMS, *State Medicaid and CHIP Income Eligibility Standards Effective January 1, 2014*, October 24, 2013.)

[79] States' decisions are based on CRS's monitoring of state activity through media outlets and state tracking of decisions done by CMS, State Refor(u)m, the Kaiser Family Foundation, the Advisory Board Company, and Avalere.

[80] U.S. Census Bureau, American Community Survey, 2012; Medicaid and CHIP Payment and Access Commission, *Report to the Congress on Medicaid and CHIP*, March 2013.

[81] In general, exchanges offer comprehensive coverage that meets the standards to be certified as "qualified health plans" (QHPs), provided it meets requirements related to marketing, choice of providers, plan networks, and other features, or is recognized by each exchange through which such plan is offered. In addition, all QHPs are required to comply with benefit, cost-sharing, and generosity components of the essential health benefits package (described above). In addition to qualified health plans, exchanges also offer multi-state QHPs, child-only QHPs, and CO-OP QHPs.

[82] "Health Policy Brief: Premium Assistance in Medicaid," *Health Affairs*, June 6, 2013.

[83] State Refor(u)m, *Governors Address Medicaid Expansion in "State of the State" Speeches*, March 2013.

[84] The definition of minimum essential coverage is broad. It includes Medicare Part A, Medicaid, the State Children's Health Insurance Program (CHIP), Tricare, the TRICARE for Life program, the veteran's health care program, the Peace Corps program, a government plan (local, state, federal) including the Federal Employees Health Benefits Program (FEHBP) and any plan established by an Indian tribal government, any plan offered in the individual, small group or large group market, a grandfathered health plan, and any other health benefits coverage, such as a state health benefits risk pool, as recognized by the Secretary of HHS in coordination with the Treasury Secretary.

[85] Genevieve M. Kenney, Lisa Dubay, Stephen Zuckerman, and Michael Huntress, *Opting Out of the Medicaid Expansion under the ACA: How Many Uninsured Adults Would not Be Eligible for Medicaid?*, The Urban Institute Health Policy Center, July 5, 2012; Benjamin D. Sommers and Arnold M. Epstein, "Perspective: Why States Are So Miffed about Medicaid - Economics, Politics, and the "Woodwork Effect"," *The New England Journal of Medicine*, vol. 365, no. 2, pp. 100-102 (July 14, 2011).

[86] The employer penalty was supposed to go into effect in 2014, but on July 2, 2013, the Obama Administration announced that it is delaying, until 2015, the enforcement and associated reporting requirements related to the employer penalty. For more information about the delay to the employer penalty, see CRS Report R43150, *Delay in Implementation of Potential Employer Penalties Under ACA*, by Bernadette Fernandez and Annie L. Mach.

[87] A "large employer" is defined in the ACA (as related to the employer penalty) as an employer who employed an average of at least 50 full-time equivalent employees (FTEs) on business days during the preceding calendar year.

[88] For more information about the employer penalty, see CRS Report R41159, *Potential Employer Penalties Under the Patient Protection and Affordable Care Act (ACA)*, by Julie M. Whittaker.

[89] Toluse Olorunnipa, "Obamacare Cutbacks Shut Hospitals Where Medicaid Went Unexpanded," *Bloomberg Government*, November 25, 2013. Letter from the Republican Governors Public Policy Committee to President Barack Obama dated July 10, 2012, available at http://www.scribd.com/doc/99730375/Medicaid-and-Exchange-Letter-Final. Sarah Kliff, "The super wonky reason states may join the Medicaid expansion," *The Washington Post*, July 8, 2012. Bob Neal, The Fiscal and Economic Impacts of Medicaid Expansion in Mississippi, 2014-2025, Mississippi Public Universities University Research Center, October 2012.

[90] This enrollment figure is measured by individuals who were "ever enrolled" in the Medicaid program throughout the year. (Medicaid and CHIP Payment and Access Commission, *Report to Congress on Medicaid and CHIP*, June 2013.)

[91] Also qualifying for Medicare are persons who have End-Stage Renal Disease (ESRD). For more information about the Medicare program, see CRS Report R40425, *Medicare Primer*.

[92] The common Medicaid eligibility pathways for Medicare beneficiaries are Supplemental Security Income (SSI) cash assistance, poverty, medically needy, special income rules for nursing home residents, home and community based services waivers, Qualified Medicare Beneficiaries, Specified Low-Income Medicare Beneficiaries, Qualified Disabled Work Individuals, and Qualifying Individuals.

[93] This expenditure figure includes both federal and state Medicaid expenditures. (Medicaid and CHIP Payment and Access Commission, *Report to Congress on Medicaid and CHIP*, June 2013.)

[94] Congressional Budget Office, *Dual-Eligible Beneficiaries of Medicare and Medicaid: Characteristics, Health Care Spending, and Evolving Policies*, June 2013.

[95] The aggregate amount of the ACA fee, to be collected across all covered insurers, will be $8.0 billion in 2014, $11.3 billion in 2015 and 2016, $13.9 billion in 2017, and $14.3 billion in 2018. After 2018, the aggregate fee will be indexed to the overall rate of annual premium growth, as calculated by the Internal Revenue Service. (For more information about the annual fee on health insurers, see CRS Report R43225, *Patient Protection and Affordable Care Act: Annual Fee on Health Insurers*, by Suzanne M. Kirchhoff.)

[96] The following are other types of health insurers or insurance arrangements not subject to the fee: entities that fully self-insure, government-run insurance programs, voluntary employees' beneficiary associations, and student health insurance coverage that educational institutions purchase through a separate, unrelated insurer.

[97] Marwood Group, *Impact of the Annual Health Insurance Tax on State Medicaid Programs*, Prepared for Molina and Amerigroup, October 2011.

[98] Ralph Giacobbe, Chris Carter, and Allison Ryne, et al., *Managed Care: Health Insurance Tax - The $8B Question*, Credit Suisse, November 8, 2013.

[99] American Academy of Actuaries, Practice Note, "Actuarial Certification of Rates for Medicaid Managed Care Programs," 2005, http://www.actuary.org/pdf/practnotes/health_medicaid_05.pdf.

[100] Ralph Giacobbe, Chris Carter, and Allison Ryne, et al., *Managed Care: Health Insurance Tax - The $8B Question*, Credit Suisse, November 8, 2013.

[101] As measured by the National Bureau of Economic Analysis.

[102] Vernon K. Smith, Robin Rudowitz, and Laura Snyder, *Medicaid in a Historic Time of Transformation: Results form a 50-State Medicaid Budget Survey for State Fiscal Years 2013 and 2014*, Kaiser Commission on Medicaid and the Uninsured, October 2013.

[103] For more information on the potential implications for these individuals, see CRS Report R42978, *Comparing Medicaid and Exchanges: Benefits and Costs for Individuals and Families*.

[104] In July 2012, the Congressional Budget Office estimated that for the average person who does not enroll in Medicaid as a result of their state not implementing the ACA Medicaid expansion and enrolls in an exchange instead, estimated federal spending will rise by roughly $3,000 in 2022—the difference between estimated additional exchange subsidies of about $9,000 and estimated Medicaid savings of roughly $6,000. (Congressional Budget Office, *Estimates for the Insurance Coverage Provisions of the Affordable Care Act Updated for the Recent Supreme Court Decision*, July 2012).

[105] The poverty guidelines (also referred to as the federal poverty level) are a version of the federal poverty measure. They are issued each year in the *Federal Register* by the Department of Health and Human Services (HHS). The guidelines are a simplification of the poverty thresholds for use for administrative purposes—for instance, determining financial eligibility for certain federal programs.

INDEX

D

E

F

G

H

I

L

M

N

O

P

R

S